TOUCHED BY
A NURSE™

Special Moments That Transform Lives

TOUCHED BY A NURSE™

Special Moments That Transform Lives

Jim Kane, MN, RN, CS, CNAA
Director, Psychiatric Liaison Services
Scripps Mercy Hospital
San Diego, CA

Carmen Germaine Warner, MSN, RN, FAAN
Nurse Consultant
San Diego, CA

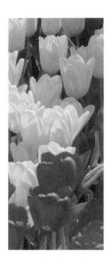
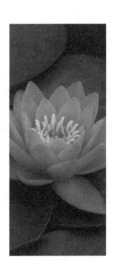
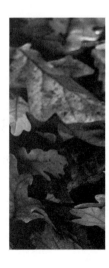
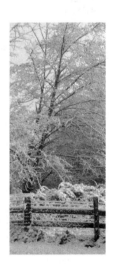

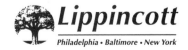

Lippincott
Philadelphia · Baltimore · New York

Acquisitions Editor: Lisa R. Marshall
Assistant Editor: Fran B. Rosen, MA, RN
Editorial Assistants: Tara Foss, Kathleen Mowery
Associate Managing Editor: Barbara Ryalls
Senior Production Manager: Helen Ewan
Production Coordinator: Patricia McCloskey
Design Coordinator: Susan Hermansen
Cover Designer: Joan Wendt

9 8 7 6 5 4 3 2 1

Library of Congress Cataloging-in-Publication Data

Kane, Jim, RN.
    Touched by a nurse™: special moments that transform lives / Jim
Kane, Carmen Germaine Warner.
        p.   cm.
    ISBN 0–7817–1873–2 (alk. paper)
    1. Nursing—Anecdotes.   2. Nurses--Anecdotes.   I. Warner, Carmen
Germaine, 1941– .   II. Title.
RT82.K327   1999
610.73—dc21
DLC
for Library of Congress   99–12590
                                                                      CIP

This *Touched By A Nurse*™ collection of vignettes uses the *Touched By A Nurse*™ trademark by permission from the owner of the trademark, James Kane, RN. Further information is available at: www.touchedbyanurse.com.

To Thom
His faith, hope, and unconditional love
made this happen
–jk

To John, my husband, and Ryan and
Tracy, our children,
Who have deeply touched this nurse
–cgw

PREFACE

"The whole is greater than the sum of the parts..."
–Martha Rogers, Nursing Theorist

Why a book of stories? Nurses are the heart and healing of our health care system. Individually and collectively, they make up an incredibly powerful healing force. As every nurse knows and this book describes, being a nurse extends far beyond the confines of a structured role or building. Nursing is more than a job.

Nurses are becoming an endangered species. A nursing shortage is predicted early in the next century. It is starting now. Health care reform, job reengineering, and managed care all have contributed to reduced financial support for care. Reimbursement for the 'value' of nursing is based on a diagnosis, regardless of the complexity of nursing care required. These factors have contributed to a reduction in registered nurse staffing, resulting in turn in a sometimes unbearable level of stress, doubt, and loss of meaning in the work. Youth are appropriately hesitant to embrace a profession of caring about others, without assurance of adequate quality and care for their own life.

Yet the lessons nurses can share are powerful, universal, and classic. Nurses have incredible stories of relationships with their patients. The primary purpose of this book is to illustrate the power of the intense healing connections that occur because of nursing. These lessons are valuable for everyone, and can promote a collective respect for the essential role that nurses fill in health care.

A second purpose is to support nurses now. During this time of revolution in health care, nurses can heal themselves by remembering their stories and having them heard. This collection of healing stories provides a source of pride and power, reminding nurses of the incredible value and purpose of their work.

This book is the combined work of my coeditor Carmen Germaine Warner and myself. She was an inspiration and a support. While she insisted that I write this preface alone, she has always been at my side. The self-appointed supporter of all potential nurse publishers, Carmen had encouraged me to write for many years. Over time I realized that the only book I wanted to do was one that would capture nurses' stories and describe what we do. And so, with Carmen's help, **Touched By A Nurse**™, the book, was born.

Soliciting story contributions began in late 1997. We approached the outstanding nurses we knew from our careers; added to the list by contacting our respective nursing organizations, boards and agencies; and, ultimately, heard from nurses all over the world. Unanimously, nurses were supportive of the idea. All contributions can be traced to someone who had a direct contact with either Carmen or myself. Despite our desire to use a story from every contributor, we had more vignettes than we could use for this edition.

We decided that each story would be entitled with the name of a person or persons in the nurse's care. All authors were asked to change names and ensure that the confidentiality of their patients was protected.

We were aware of the many types of nursing roles and were concerned that our book would be balanced to illustrate these roles. Yet we consciously made no specific effort to elicit stories from any specific settings or roles. These are stories of the human experience.

As the vignettes for the book arrived from the contributors, I came to cherish the mission this book represents. Truly, the whole is greater than the sum of the parts. Every nurse who wrote a story remembered an event of the heart, an event of healing to share. These are deeply personal and moving accounts of a global profession that is unified by care and love. Most of these stories have never been told. It became a sacred trust to play a role in having nurses' stories told.

My life was changed because I became a nurse. I hope that other lives will be changed as a result of reading this book, and that all readers are **Touched By A Nurse**™.

Thank you for caring about what nurses do. There is nothing else like it in the world.

Jim Kane

ACKNOWLEDGMENTS

Clearly a work of this sort is not the achievement of one or two people, but many. This book would not have happened had it not been for a group of devoted nurses, who thoughtfully shared their personal work in the form of their stories. There were no promises when the contributors first submitted their stories, yet the result reflects works from the heart. This book would have not happened without the caring of our nurse authors.

In addition to the contributors, many people helped with many parts of the book, and must be mentioned. These nurses and non-nurses believed in this project and helped to assure the completion of the book in every way, from editing to mailing letters. They continue providing unconditional love. They are listed here alphabetically since all have been indispensable in some way: Susan Allison (the Nyack connection), Karen Bauer, Thom Birkenstock, Jill Bormann, Rita Callahan, Colin Crawford, Josh Ellis, Tony Ellis, Jackie Flaskerud, Jerry Gold, Rev. Kathy Hearn, Ann Kelly, Ken Knara, Nick McCarter, Pam Minarik (the Asian and Nyack connections), Jane Neese, Gloria Nocon, Gale Osborn, Lori Perry, Jodi Porter, Clark Ritter, Ryan Robbins, Michael Scahill, Thelma Schor, Johnette Thomas, Daniel Travert, Evelyn Virrey, Kurt Williams, and Nancy Woods.

Special thanks to the team at Lippincott Williams & Wilkins, to our editor Lisa Marshall, and to Fran Rosen for her warrior style and wit.

It goes without saying that the professional friendship that started this project has grown over the years into a powerful mutual respect and caring between coauthors. The support for each other was critical to all parts of the book.

CONTENTS

TOUCHED BY
A NURSE™

Special Moments That Transform Lives

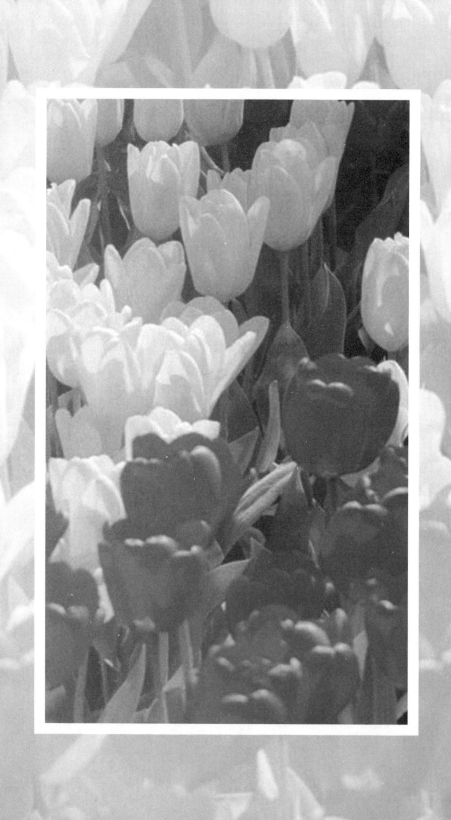

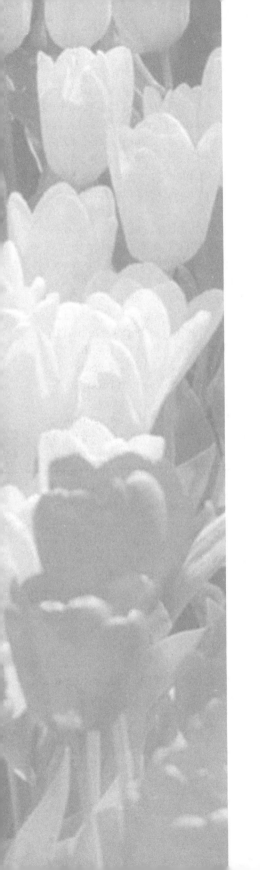

HOPE

RICHARD

In the spring of 1997, I volunteered for California AIDS Ride 4 to help support the 2,500 riders who rode their bicycles 560 miles from San Francisco to Los Angeles and raised more than 9 million dollars to benefit California AIDS organizations.

Our team provided riders with various medical treatments, from minor sprains and abrasions to AIDS-related illnesses. We set up our 25-bed hospital tent in a different city every day, and provided treatment from early afternoon till midnight, when the tent closed. Each night one of us was on standby for emergencies.

The 3rd day took the cyclists inland through the central San Joaquin valley. The temperature rose to almost 90°. Despite constant reminders to drink lots of water, many riders became dehydrated. That evening we saw almost 50 people with dizziness, nausea and exhaustion—classic signs of dehydration. Within 3 hours we started more than 30 IVs, and by midnight we had administered almost 80 liters of IV fluid.

One of the riders who came to the tent that night was Richard. Because he was too weak to walk, he was almost dragged in by two of his friends. Richard was in the advanced stage of AIDS. He had trained for the ride for almost a year and had raised more than $3000. But this day's 70-mile trip in hot weather had completely depleted his resources. He was hypotensive and had a slight fever.

That night, when he was lying on the stretcher and as I started the IV, tears were running down his face. I could see he felt miserable and was totally exhausted. He took my hand and with a desperate look asked me to help him to get better. He had to finish this ride. He told me that his lover had passed away 2 years before, and that he had promised to do this ride in his memory.

It was late and the tent started to empty out. I was sitting at Richard's side and we talked for a long time. After I hung the third liter of fluid, I could see the color coming back to Richard's face. His fever was gone and he was drinking liquids—he felt much better. Richard went back to his tent. In the morning, he had to get rechecked. Without that, he would not be able to get his bike back. His blood pressure was good and he had just finished a big breakfast—he was ready to go.

Three days later I saw Richard as one of the first of the 2500 riding into the closing ceremony in L.A. Tears were again streaming down his face, but this time he looked like the happiest man alive. When he saw me, he came up to me and gave me a big hug. "I made it," he said. "Thank you very much." ∎

Jürgen Deutzer, RN
1997

4

INMATE
SUPPORT
GROUP

I was one of several psychiatric mental health RNs who were initiating a research project with women in the Michigan State Prison System. We had been funded by the National Institute of Drug Abuse to provide substance abuse group counseling. The goals of the project were to assist chemically dependent women to become clean and sober and to maintain recovery after release. The constructs of the Personalized Nursing Model were simple: identify the focal concerns of these women and make every effort to assist them with their needs.

The first session, with 15 to 20 inmates, was on a blustery March Michigan day. I had arrived in plenty of time to make it through the complex entry process. There were papers to sign, belongings to be searched, and locked gates and doors to slow one's progress every step of the way. I awaited my colleagues eagerly, unaware that they had been delayed because they had stopped to take a forbidden photo on the way into the prison grounds. While I was waiting, the guards began to usher the silent inmates into the room. As the minutes ticked by, I was acutely aware that these women were with

me, not only because they had a drug or alcohol problem, but also because they had committed various criminal acts. With the guards standing by outside the room, I began to make eye contact with women who had committed armed and unarmed robbery, credit card fraud, larceny, probation violations, assault, prostitution, possession and sale of illegal substances, and manslaughter. They ranged in age from 19 to 45 and though some were from elsewhere in Michigan, the majority were African American women from Detroit's inner city.

I felt isolated, uncomfortable, and was fearful for my own safety. I wondered how I might relate to women so different in ethnic background and life experience from myself. What could I offer them that hadn't already been learned on the streets? The responsibility seemed overwhelming, but I took a deep breath and began. I shared information about the project and myself. I offered the hope that each of the women in that room could make a better life for herself, that each had a right and an ability to feel good about herself and her capabilities. I was there to help them believe in and achieve their dreams. The women began speaking up, with soft voices initially. As they began to talk about themselves, their voices became stronger. They looked at me and at each other. The atmosphere became charged.

They began to ask questions. I met Nancy, a 34-year-old mother of two children whom the court wanted to remove from her care. She experienced disabling migraines and worried about her sick mother. Nancy was so afraid of losing her children. Marcella told me of her heroin addiction, of her worries about her physical health, her depression and anger, and her inability to cope with treatment by others in the prison. Lucy told me of her uterine cancer that had not yet been treated, of shoplifting each day to support her mother's cocaine habit. Lucy told me she would do anything to help her mother, even though she herself was only 19 years old. She had prostituted herself for drug money. Denette had been physically and verbally abused all her life, first by her father, then her stepfather, and now she was in an abusive relationship. Marcie expressed a desire to learn how to better parent her children, 5 years, 20 months, and 10 months old. Vanessa wanted a job but said no one wanted her, especially now that she had a prison record. She did not much care whether she went on living.

As the humanness, experiences, vulnerabilities, and strengths of these women became apparent, I found my fears rapidly evaporating. Before me arose a challenge. Might I help these women move, painfully at times, step by step, toward a life that perhaps few of them dared envision? Were they willing to strive for a life with opportunities to feel good about themselves, where they could identify real job skills or learn to balance a checkbook? Would they choose to learn parenting skills, to practice ways of staying clean and sober, to redefine the relationships in which they had been involved? There was hope of a life outside of these prison walls where others, including my absent colleagues, would be there to offer support, guidance, and a safety net in the face of risk, relapse, or failure.

I would share with these women the knowledge, attitudes, and experiences that I carry with me as a nurse: the warmth, caring, and support they needed, the recognition that dreams can be realized, and that the desire to change is the key that will open many doors.

They, in turn, had already revealed to me the strength of their human spirits, their ability to stand strong, speak out, and their desire to start over, despite the most adverse circumstances. They had shared the gift of love for their families that flourished and grew despite addiction, incarceration, and the constraints of time and distance. They, too, had hopes and dreams, and together we began to make them real. ∎

Sandy Gunderson
Goldsmith, MSN, RN, CS
1986

JIM

On the cardiothoracic surgical unit, our census of CT patients usually dwindled by the weekend. I was not surprised when I came into work one Saturday and found that I was assigned to an 18-year-old 'off service' trauma patient. As I received report, I learned that Jim, a diabetic, had been involved in a motor vehicle accident the previous afternoon. Among his injuries was a facial fracture that had placed pressure onto his optic nerve. During the night he had been rushed back to the OR in an attempt to relieve the impingement and save his sight.

Jim was still intubated and rather sleepy, but hemodynamically he was stable. I went about my normal routine, talking quietly to Jim, explaining what I was doing, as I assessed him. He followed simple commands, but his pupils were dilated and unresponsive to light, just as I had been told in the report. He appeared to fall back to sleep as soon as he was left alone.

As the day progressed, Jim had many visitors, including all the teams of physicians who were caring for him. First the trauma service checked his pupils, then the neuro service, and finally, ophthalmology. They all asked him if he was able to see the light they showed him. Jim would shake his head no, and they would walk away without a further word to him. No one offered any explanation. By the time the third team had seen him, he was much more awake. The unit was calm and quiet. I decided to sit down and talk to Jim. Pulling a chair up to his bedside, I gently took his hand and asked if he knew where he was. He nodded. I asked if he knew why. "No." I told him he had been in a car accident and asked if he wanted to know his injuries, which he did. I started by telling him about his leg fracture, his splenectomy, and his broken ribs. Then I told him that he had fractured some bones in his face and that the doctors were shining a light in his eyes because they had operated to remove a bone fragment that had put pressure on the nerves to his eyes. The doctors hoped that his sight would return when the swelling went down. He squeezed my hand and mouthed "thank you," and we sat there quietly for a few minutes.

Later that day I met Jim's mother. She told me all about how he had just moved out on his own and was attending the local junior college part-time and working. She told me also about the accident. The theory was that Jim had had some type of hypo- or hyperglycemic reaction and blacked out. We stood and talked outside his door for awhile. She said quietly that she couldn't tell Jim about his eyes. I encouraged her to sit at Jim's bedside and just visit with him.

They sat together for an hour and held hands.

The next day Jim was ready to be extubated. As soon as the tube was out, he starting reaching out and managed to grab my arm. I assured him that he was hoarse because of the tube, but he said "No, no, were you my nurse yesterday?" "Yes" I replied. "I thought I recognized your voice. Thank you so much. You were the only person who would say anything to me about my sight. No one said a word after they asked me if I could see the light. But you did. And you stayed with me."

Jim's mother arrived shortly after he was extubated. She was standing outside the room, afraid to come in. She asked "What do I say?" "Just tell him the truth, that you love him and that you're here for him." She hugged me tight and again I cried, this time with her.

By the next shift, Jim had been transferred to a general nursing floor. I never saw Jim or his mother again, but I will always remember him when I try to explain how nursing is different than medicine, and why I am proud to be a nurse. ∎

Barb McGurgan, MSN, RN, CCRN
1994

MAMA

Our 17-member group, OPERATION BLESSING MEDICAL STRIKE FORCE TEAM 5 arrived on September 21, 1994 in Goma, a small town on the Zaire–Rwandan border, where more than one million Rwandan refugees had set up camp in the foothills of a still-active volcano mountain range. We would help out daily at the hospital, where many refugees had been admitted with shrapnel and bullet wounds, burns and fractures. Kibumba camp was a sight of total devastation. Makeshift shelters and improvised shacks were everywhere. Women were cooking on open fires, men were standing, smoking, or selling contraband items, and thousands of children roamed.

The Director of Nurses of the Goma Hospital opened the door to the women's surgical ward. Fourteen pairs of deep hollow eyes stared at us in wasted, malnourished bodies. "Our electricity came on late this morning, so we are still waiting for our instruments to be sterilized" said Paluka, the Zairian medical student who served as our interpreter. We went from bed to bed, greeting each patient and trying to communicate through sign language and the interpreter. With the frequent warning "Please be careful" still ringing in my ears, I

surreptitiously put on my gloves. But by the third bed I felt ashamed of myself. How would these people open up to me if I did not even want to touch them ungloved? So I slipped off my gloves, hoping it would go unnoticed.

Then I saw her, a face full of pain and suffering, eyes begging "Help me!" A repelling, distinct odor came from her bed. She was lying supine on the bare plastic of her mattress. "Bomb wound" offered Paluka when he saw the question in my eyes. "I just can't take it anymore" said a team nurse, who disappeared with the interpreter. The woman on the bed locked her eyes into mine, wordlessly begging, anxious to see what I could do.

"O Lord, help me! Where do I start—the odor is so overwhelming!" my heart screamed silently. In my broken kinyanRwandan, I tried: "Muraho Mama" (Good morning, Mama—Mama is a form of respect). No response. I tried again, now from the depth of my heart. "Imana Igufashe" (God bless you). Her eyes softened a little. Tenderly, I started to clean her wound. Mama started to wail and mumble. "What is she saying?" I asked Paluka. "She is praying out loud" he said. Mama closed her eyes, tired from the lengthy procedure. I held her hand for a long time, communicating by touch. This was just a droplet in the bucket; there was so little I could do.

Every morning Mama's eyes were calling me when I opened the door to the ward. Her medical record revealed that she was on antibiotics but on no pain medications at all. "Can we ask the doctor to give her some pain medications before we start with her dressings?" I asked Paluka. "We do not have any" he replied. When we stocked our medical supply kit that night, I bargained for a box of Anacin tablets. Armed with a whole box of surgical dressing kits, thick masks, and my Anacin, we started off another day of wound dressings, this time also in the men's ward and overflow tents. Smiles of thankfulness beamed on the faces of those who endured so much pain. "Your heart has too much pity" was Paluka's comment on my Anacin campaign. "The people of Africa are strong."

Mama did not wail so loudly during dressing changes. The pain medication had the necessary effect, but she kept on mumbling her prayers. "Merci" she would say afterwards, her eyes bathed in thankfulness.

This experience with the Rwandan refugees changed my life. I know that as a nurse, I can daily listen, touch, encourage, help those who hurt, and I can give the kind of loving support that is needed. ∎

Debbie DenBoer, RN, BSN,
CGRN
1994

MARIAN

I was not a nurse at the time of my son's birth and did not complete my nursing education until some years later. When I specialized in the field of infection prevention and control a few years later, one of my first goals was to examine 'rituals and magic' in the control of infection and eliminate those with no scientific basis. Infection prevention and control rituals surrounding childbirth were some of the first to be questioned as the natural childbirth movement picked up momentum, and gradually they were eliminated as my colleagues and I evaluated their lack of scientific validity. Today I have a world view of infection prevention and control, but it was not always that way.

My son Gar was born at 7:00 pm on a Monday evening, November 1968, in a small-town hospital in Mississippi. He was delivered by the only obstetrician in town, and came into the world with a head full of dark hair, fists clenched, and yelling loudly. He was 2 weeks past due and his father and grandparents were eagerly standing by in the waiting room to find out if the new baby was a boy or girl.

During the delivery, the obstetrician kindly positioned a mirror so I could watch. However, Gar's father was not allowed into the inner sanctum of the delivery room and was told he could not touch his son until the two of us were discharged home from the hospital the following Saturday. The rationale for this was that if anyone except the mother, the physician, and the hospital staff touched the baby, the infant would be contaminated with organisms that could bring infection into the nursery. Of course, the physician and hospital staff interacted with many people other than new mothers and infants during work, but the nursery staff changed into special clothing. Physicians and other hospital staff put on cover gowns to enter the nursery. This clothing was intended to provide a "clean, infection-free" environment for infants in the nursery. Fathers and other family could visit the mother in her room when the infant was safely in the nursery, but could only view the infant through the nursery windows. Like many rules, these had been in effect for years and were rarely questioned by anyone.

On Tuesday afternoon, my nurse for the evening shift was a middle-aged woman from England named Marian. As she was checking on my progress and straightening my bed, she told me that she had been a midwife in England before moving to the United States with her husband, who was in the military. Her husband was stationed at a nearby military base, and she was working in this hospital as an LVN because she could not be an RN in the United States without additional education, and Mississippi offered no opportunities for nurse midwives. I told her how sad my husband was not to be able to hold his new son, that he had waited until his late 30s to have his first child, and was very eager to begin the bonding process. Marian went to the door, looked up and down the hall, and closed the door carefully. She came over to my bed and whispered softly, "I know how important it is for fathers to bond with their infants. And, I could lose my job over this, but if you'll tell your husband to come up the back stairs at 10:00 tonight, I'll meet him and let him hold his son. Please don't tell anybody. I really could lose my job over this."

My husband came to visit at 7:00 that evening. I asked him to close the door and I whispered instructions for 10:00 pm in his ear.

The next day during morning visiting hours he came into my room beaming ear to ear, "he's so tiny and so soft, and so wonderful..." and continued with a stream of excited words about his first 'unofficial' visit with his new son.

On Saturday, when the day nurse 'officially' let Gar's dad touch him, once I was seated in the car with him in my lap (before the days of mandatory car seats), he made appropriate joyful comments about touching his son 'for the first time.' So far as I know, none of the hospital officials ever knew that Marian let some dads come up the back stairs late at night to bond with their new infants. It was a wonderful gift she gave us, and we have never forgotten her kindness and willingness to break the rule that didn't make much sense to her or to us. ∎

Marguerite McMillan Jackson,
PhD, RN, FAAN
1998

CHARLES

My 3rd year with the home health oncology team, the Administrative Director for the agency approached me to request a favor. She explained that her first boss in home health was seriously ill with liver cancer. "I would appreciate if you would take the case and manage it through its entirety." I knew I would have to perform at my very best on this high-profile case, and I wanted to be 100% sucessful.

Charles Green was a 39-year-old owner of his business. I remember thinking, "He and I are the same age—this could be me." Only 6 months before, Charles had been diagnosed with a highly invasive form of liver cancer. He had already experienced surgery, extensive radiation therapy, some chemotherapy, and was now trying numerous supportive cancer treatments. Mrs. Green had thoroughly involved herself in all levels of her husband's care. Charles was not very religious but began to gain insight into his spiritual belief.

One day, after returning to the office, I spoke with the Administrative Director. I said, "I can't do this, I'm not sure I am the right nurse for this patient and family." "I believe in you, both personally and professionally. You are the right nurse for them," she replied. It was important for Charles and I to talk.

He stated, "I am getting tired." I asked, "Are you afraid of dying?" "No," he replied. "I am afraid of the actual process. I don't want to suffer." As he lay in bed, I pulled up close to him and leaned forward. Holding his hand I said, "The goals are to keep you within your home, and keep you as comfortable as possible, which includes controlling the pain." We agreed to the goals. All of my caring, skill, and knowledge would be spent accomplishing the goals. Mrs. Green agreed.

Charles soon discontinued all treatments, which had become exhausting and cumbersome, with no positive medical change in his status. It would be just a matter of time. My pager was always on.

It was two o'clock in the morning when I received the page. I arrived in time to assist with Charles's final needs. Our goals had been met. His family surrounded Charles. "Finally, coming face to face with my own mortality has been such an incredibly transformational event that I cannot describe it. It is literally beyond my ability at this point to put into words the spiritual and emotional roller coaster which I am on, and which has so significantly changed me." Before his death, he looked around the room and said, "WOW!" I said good-bye to Charles and his family. ∎

Rita R. Callahan, MA, RN
1993

MR. DU'S TAI-TAI

I was making rounds with two head nurses at a large psychiatric hospital north of Beijing.

We had visited a 40-year-old man who was transferred from a general hospital. Mr. Du was diagnosed with 'hysteria' as evidenced by a nonpathologic paralysis of his lower extremities. He had been severely beaten and was suffering from post-traumatic stress syndrome.

Mr. Du was a friendly man who openly welcomed our weekly visits. His Tai-Tai (wife) was always present. She stayed with him throughout his hospitalizations. There was no sign of a wheelchair in his room or close by. Upon inquiring, I found that Du Tai-Tai, not a large person, carried her husband on her back to wherever he needed to be, on the ward and off. This form of transport was surprising only to me. It was accepted by her husband and the nursing staff.

At our interviews, I noticed that Du Tai-Tai sat quietly, offering input only when encouraged to do so. On one occasion, when asking Mr. Du, "How do you think your illness is affecting your family?" I glanced towards his wife and noticed a look

Kathleen Ann DeGrazia, MA, BSN, RN
1998

of pain on her face. Du Tai-Tai made no comment and looked towards the floor while her husband gave a nebulous response to the question.

At my next visit, Mr. Du was sleeping and his wife was diligently sitting there with him, giving a perfect opportunity for me to talk with her and focus on the family. Du Tai-Tai was most willing to talk with us and gladly received the chance to be out of the room.

In our interview, we had learned that the doctors explained very little to Mr. Du about his illness. Du Tai-Tai revealed that she knew little and was apprehensive about either asking her husband any questions, or revealing how she was feeling. She was also concerned about her elderly in-laws.

On a piece of paper, I drew a circle and attached four small circles to it. I identified the main circle as her, the others being her physical husband, the illness, the family, and her own concerns. I then said, "It seems to me that you not only carry your husband physically on your back, but you also carry the emotional burdens of the illness, family and yourself." Looking straight at her, I first saw a small tear, but then a smile and a nod of her head. For the first time, someone acknowledged the impact of the illness for her. At that one moment I connected with Du Tai-Tai. I could not take away the realities of her husband's illness, but I could acknowledge the burden she carried. This acknowledgment seemed to make the difference to her. ∎

RANDY

During my senior year of nursing school, our family lost our 3½-year-old brother, Robbie, to acute lymphocytic leukemia. Because of this painful experience, I thought I would never be able to care for children.

However, 5 years later, the director of nursing at a hospital in Florida where I was practicing, asked me to accept a nurse manager position in pediatrics. I accepted the challenge to do the best job I could.

A year after assuming the nurse manager role, a 10-year-old boy named Randy was admitted, diagnosed with acute lymphocytic leukemia. Robbie, my brother, would have been about the same age. During the next year and a half, along with multiple staff, we coordinated Randy's care and provided support to his parents, brother and sister.

One event was especially meaningful to Randy, his family, and to me. At the time, home care was generally reserved for convalescence or terminal illness and used little technology. One weekend I received a call from Randy's mother informing me that Randy's IV had become dislodged. She asked me if I would restart his IV since none of the nurses who were on duty were known by Randy. He was very apprehensive about this procedure and felt like a guinea pig with multiple venapunctures. I contacted Randy's attending physician and discussed the circumstances. About an hour later, Randy and his parents came to my home, where I had obtained the necessary equipment and restarted his IV. Randy and his parents were so appreciative that I had been responsive to assist him.

As Randy's illness advanced, on one hospitalization not long before his death, he asked to talk with me. He was honest and direct, expressing his feelings of tiredness with all the various types of therapies he had experienced. He wanted to stop this and he was concerned about how his parents would react. After listening to him and reflecting on his questions, we had a lengthy discussion. Then, I suggested that he speak with his parents and share his feelings about what he wanted in the way of care and his desires about his life.

Shortly after that, Randy died. His parents later expressed their appreciation for the care I had given to their son. It was a defining moment in my professional practice as well as my personal growth, that I was able to provide care and also heal at the same time from my own personal loss. ∎

Mary Lou Helfrich Jones,
PhD, RN, CNAA
1971

BESS

I had been a registered nurse for 1 year when I accepted a staff nurse position on a 24-bed head and neck surgical oncology unit. Although I had not initially requested that specialty when I interviewed for the job, I was excited about the challenges that I would encounter.

Some of the nurses who specialized in eye, ear, nose, and minor throat disorders said, "Oh...how can you work with those patients? All those tracheotomies, mucus, and odors? Isn't it sad what they do to those people?"

Needless to say, I began to doubt my new assignment. Although I prided myself on my nursing skills, I began to question my decision. I asked myself, could I do it?

When I started the clinical portion of the orientation, I was teamed with an experienced nurse on the unit. I was to observe her as she cared for her patients and assist her until I felt comfortable. That morning in report, the night nurse described a patient called Bess.

Bess was a 65-year-old woman who had recently undergone extensive surgery for cancer of her nasal cavity, palate, and related facial structures. Since the cancer had invaded much of the central portion of her face, Bess was left with an enormous disfigured area that had been grafted.

I had a quick glimpse of Bess in her private room at the end of the hallway during one of the unit tours. In addition to having a tracheotomy tube, feeding equipment, and IV lines in place, Bess wore several 4x4 gauze pads loosely taped over her surgical defect. It was difficult to forget Bess's unique facial profile, even from a distance. Report was over. It was time to take care of Bess. As I entered her room with my preceptor, Bess had just finished feeding herself through a tube in her neck. She was sitting on the side of the bed, writing us a note on her magic slate. She asked us if we were ready to teach her how to do her facial wound irrigations. Although Bess seemed really eager about this procedure, I had concerns. I wondered if I could deal with seeing her disfigurement—I didn't want to grimace when I first saw her wound. Would I be effective and be able to help her deal with the change in her physical appearance? The comments made by the other nurses came back to haunt me.

My preceptor removed the gauze from Bess's face. I had never seen anything like this. There was a large opening in the middle of Bess's face that started from where the bridge of her nose used to be and continued downward across her cheeks. The entire roof of her mouth was missing. Two bright blue eyes rested at the very edge of the defect, and I could see the base of her brain and pulsating tissue within the cavernous wound.

It was as though Bess sensed my hesitation. Using her magic slate, she began to tell me what the surgery had meant to her, about the unbearable pain she had experienced before the surgery, and how comfortable she felt now. She boasted of her grandchildren and told me how she loved being with them. Bess wrote that, before surgery, she would tape gauze to her face, covering the cancer. The bandages frightened her grandchildren and made her feel bad. She told me that she looked forward to the time when her surgical wound would be healed. At that time, she would be fitted with a facial prosthesis to cover her defect. She felt that her grandchildren would react much better to the prosthesis than to the gauze. Then she could enjoy them once again.

During the next several weeks, I witnessed Bess's dreams come true. She eventually received her facial prosthesis, along with an oral piece that enabled her to talk and eat by mouth. She was proficient in her self-care activities and was discharged to her home with her grandchildren. Bess went on with the rest of her life.

Twenty-five years later, as I continue to be involved in the specialty of head and neck cancer nursing, I often reflect back to my experience with Bess as a new nurse, and remember what Bess taught me. It is important to ask yourself, "What does this experience mean to the patient and family?" Bess was comfortable with her decision. Why shouldn't I have been comfortable with it too? ∎

Joan Such Lockhart, PhD, RN,
CORLN
1973

BILL

Just the sound of the word 'trauma' can make your heart start racing, as your tired legs spring into action with a renewed energy that carries body and mind into the anticipated realm of what we emergency nurses affectionately call "organized chaos." The trauma room comes to life as noises pervade the air.

The staff are costumed in plastic aprons, rubber gloves, giant goggles, face masks, shoe covers. As we wait, a quiet sets over the room. Everyone is lost in their own thoughts. We have every piece of equipment that we own within our reach so we will be ready for anything.

In the far distance the wail of the siren breaks into private thoughts. It gets louder as the paramedics race against the 'golden hour.' Too many minutes outside the hospital decreases the patient's chance for recovery.

Silent prayers are said as the back doors of the ambulance fly open. The trauma team can be heard crashing through the trauma bay doors as on the show *ER*. Eye contact is made with the paramedic. "It doesn't look good," he tells you with his eyes. "Gunshot wound to the abdomen with an unknown downtime. Looks

Kelly Jane O'Hara, BSN, RN, CEN
1997

like he lost a lot of blood," he tells you verbally. You stay focused on getting Bill out of "the bus" and into the trauma room. It's hard to stay focused when Bill is moaning loudly and the family is all around you screaming and crying. The paramedic is trying to give you a report, the police are asking you questions, and Bill's mother is clutching your arm begging you to please save her son. You finally get Bill into the trauma room and onto the stretcher. You say a silent prayer that this is one of those nights that miracles happen.

You look at the clock and realize that only 10 minutes have passed. You begin to write the play that unfolds in front of you. Hands fly back and forth over the patient. The trauma team settles into that nonverbal rhythm when all the team have the same finely tuned skills and knowledge. Your eyes flit from person to person, activity to activity.

You document observations, findings, procedures, treatment, times, places, persons, cc's, milligrams, vital signs, and then the final "transferred to OR via stretcher on monitor accompanied by RN" and sign your name. Within 20 minutes of arrival, Bill has been transferred to the OR. That night you see one of the SICU nurses and inquire about Bill. She gives you the thumbs-up sign. Yes! Another save! You finish your shift and go home. They ask you at home if anything happened at work today and you smile and reply, "Nothing out of the ordinary." ∎

SAL

I was a new grad in August 1972 and had been working on a surgical specialty unit for 6 weeks. I was 19 years old. Sal was admitted after surgery during the day shift. He was 16 years old, and had been working a construction job with his father when he fell off a high ladder. He sustained a broken spine and was paralyzed from the neck down. The prognosis was somewhat hopeful for slight recovery but bleak for full functioning. We were told he would recover some abilities over the course of a year and that it was not clearly predictable what his condition would be at the end of that time. The entire staff was particularly taken with his youth and extent of his disability. Sal came to us in a full body cast, asleep from anesthetics and pain medications. I vividly remember thinking "How awful! What a tragedy, he is so young." The reality of how close in age we were was particularly disturbing.

Sal was a great patient! He rarely complained and was almost always in a good mood. When awful and ugly medical procedures needed to be done, or routine but uncomfortable physical needs were cared for, he was quick with humor and a sense of decorum. Sal, at 16, had wisdom, wit, and style. People might think this was a 'New York' style. He was raised in Brooklyn, one of four children, to a lower-middle class, blue-collar father and homemaking mother. They were Italian Catholics. Sal said "I'm not much of a student. I like working with my Dad—as soon as he'll let me quit school I will." For 16, he seemed somewhat mature, flirtatious, and a bit precocious. He had a girlfriend who visited frequently when he was admitted, but after a few weeks, slowed her pace. His mother, father, and three sisters visited every evening initially. After a couple of months, they too slowed their visiting to once or twice a week. Sal put up a good front, but the reality of his situation was obvious to us, his caretakers and 'new' family.

I loved being a nurse. I loved working with the patients, the feeling of helping people and doing good. I loved talking with the patients. I felt a strong need to listen to them and let them share their feelings with me as they encountered physical hurdles that left them emotionally unbalanced.

Sal and I shared many moments during the long span of his inpatient stay on my unit, but New Year's Eve was special. I regularly worked the day shift, but during the holiday week Sal asked if I would work New Year's Eve. I considered his request and switched with a grateful coworker to work.

Arriving on the unit at 11 pm, I took report and found us full as usual. There were no untoward events occurring, and all patients were resting comfortably. Many would be discharged the next day. Making my first set of rounds, Sal was awake and asked me to make sure to come see him before midnight and wish him a Happy New Year. After managing my routine duties, I checked on Sal. I got back to him at midnight, after rounds. Sal smiled brightly and displayed a bottle of champagne. His father had brought him the champagne as a gift for a NEW New Year, "Make a wish" he said, "and it will come true!" Sal asked me to help wish him to walk again in the New Year. Whoa, I thought, this is not okay. Sal is underage, he's a patient under my care, he shouldn't be drinking, and it sure isn't okay for me to be drinking champagne with him. He told me I was a "fuddy-duddy," assured me he had no sleep or pain medications, and reminded me that "life is short!"

Despite my concerns, my gut told me Sal needed to do this. So, we shared one glass of champagne. I'm not sure how many more for him. We wished for his walking power.

At age 17, Sal was discharged to a rehabilitation facility. He had the ability to stand with assistance, but not yet to walk. I think of him still and hope that now he can walk. Sal taught me that my true talent is in the 'talking' field. I have worked in mental health for the past 25 years, hopefully touching others with my heart as they continue to touch me with theirs. ∎

Marlene Nadler Moodie, MSN,
RN, CS
1973

MADELYN

Two to three months after her initial diagnosis and treatment for non-Hodgkin's lymphoma, Madelyn had been receiving chemotherapy based on an aggressive but successful protocol, and the nursing staff on the medical–oncology unit was concerned. She was depressed and was being seen by the psychiatric consultation service and treated with antidepressant medication. Despite these measures, the staff believed she was suicidal because of the disturbing casual comments she interjected into conversations with her nurses. They asked if I would see her and evaluate her suicidality. Though I primarily worked with the staff, as the Psychiatric Liaison Clinical Nurse Specialist, this case seemed an exception. That's how Madelyn and I met.

In her room, the bright Florida sunshine was diffused by closed miniblinds. I observed a petite, somewhat frail, pretty young woman looking much younger than her 31 years, lying in bed. She wore a colorful scarf over her baldness and had on makeup and nail polish. This carefully constructed exterior could not camouflage her fatigue. Though keeping up normal appearances seemed to have drained what little energy she had left, I admired the will it took to do so. Even from these meager first impressions, I suspected she wasn't actively suicidal.

But I valued the nurses' clinical judgment and knew there was much to still learn about Madelyn. Madelyn was an extremely private, introverted person, who nonetheless endured the fairly intrusive questions I, a stranger, asked her. She wasn't suicidal. She was exhausted—by the treatments, by the strange environment she found so offensive, by trying to stay in control of a situation that was so out of her control. She was single, had worked as a paralegal, had a few close friends, but was closest to her sister in Tampa. As I learned in time, her parents relied more on Madelyn than she on them.

What Madelyn wanted was someone to help her figure out how to cope with her disease and all that came with it. She wanted to be understood, not badgered into a bone marrow transplant—to be treated as her previous competent self, not a helpless cancer patient. These were the things we first talked about. Since Madelyn was looking for coping strategies, I offered to help her with relaxation and visualization techniques.

We met several times before she was discharged. We set up a psychiatric nurse home visit to follow-up, but after one visit, Madelyn decided it wasn't necessary. It was several months before I saw Madelyn again. I knew she'd made an impression on me; I didn't realize how powerful it would become.

A few months later, I was making rounds in the ICU when I overheard the nurses talking about their newest patient. I was stunned when I realized their new, critically ill patient was Madelyn. After her last round of chemotherapy, she had the misfortune to end up with typhlitis (a very rare, deadly side effect—her surgeon's notes before surgery said she had 0% chance of living without surgery, 1%–2% even with it). After surgery to excise her decayed bowel, she was alive, but with a below-the-knee amputation and a colostomy. I found myself overwhelmed by distressed feelings for the entire experience of this young woman. I offered words of consolation, and outrage at all she'd gone through: "It seems like too much to bear." She seemed comforted to have her pain acknowledged and despite this pain, was glad to see me. As I was about to leave, I said "If I can be of help in any way, let me know." She asked if I would read to her. I felt embarrassingly grateful that she'd found a way for me to help her.

Madelyn and I worked together from September until her death the following March, a mere 10 months from her initial diagnosis. These were some of the most painful and rewarding months I've ever spent.

What did we do during that time? Anything that supported Madelyn. She decided to change physicians. I helped her accomplish this. She was able to negotiate routines and preferences with the nursing staff and other doctors,

with some coaching from me. I worked with the staff to help them be open to her requests. We read magazines, discussed fashion, talked about Doris Day movies and anything that took her mind off the decline of her situation. She struggled to make sense of it all— as she said once "Only bad things have happened to me since my diagnosis; why do I keep drawing only the short straws? It's all happening so quickly." She was angry as well as sad. I listened to her rail at God about her fate. I tried always to keep in mind what I learned about Madelyn that first visit—her need to feel competent and capable. Sometimes that meant she didn't want to need me either.

You might think I only had painful feelings for all the suffering Madelyn went through. That was certainly part of it. But more distressing were my own conflicted feelings. Yes, some were about her suffering, but mostly I felt conflicted about Madelyn's difficulty in allowing anyone (especially me) to help her. It might make me feel better to help her; it didn't always help her feel better. Mostly what there was to 'do' for Madelyn was to just be with her. This meant to endure along with her all of her anguish and trials.

In working with Madelyn, I needed to find a way make sense of what seemed like horrendous karma or God being on vacation indefinitely. I wrestled again with feelings I had for my Dad, whom I had taken care of at home for 6 weeks before he died from cancer. I was confronted with how hard it is for me to feel helpless. And I dealt with liking Madelyn so much that it felt too painful for me to watch her suffer. I worried that I was losing my objectivity. I consulted a trusted, wise colleague. She said that although many of my feelings were provoked by this situation, she didn't fear that I'd harmed Madelyn with them. The good and bad news was "this is it—this is what the work is all about."

Sometime in February, Madelyn finally was able to hear her doctor say nothing more could be done. It was time for comfort measures. She went home soon thereafter. We talked on the phone weekly. We made plans to have lunch. Sometimes I wrote her brief notes. She had a few radiation treatments for symptom control. She looked awful and was usually too weak to walk. While she received radiation therapy, I spent time with her sister and mother, nobody really talking much.

One day, her mother called to say Madelyn died. Maybe it was a blessing for Madelyn but it really hurt those of us still alive. I went to her funeral mass and learned there was much I still didn't know about Madelyn. She was a beloved choir member in her church and many came to acknowledge her life.

I had my own private closing for Madelyn and me in a park by my house. I cried and rode home on my bike.

All that Madelyn taught me can't be wrapped up in a neat way. I learned a lot about myself. I learned about tolerating painful feelings, my own and others', and about suffering and dying. I'm better because of this. I've outgrown the way I had made sense of loss and pain. There are few quick fixes for important things and that's okay and a relief. I recognize I need God and believe He doesn't cause bad things to happen in this world but is there to give us the strength to deal with the difficult times. I thank Madelyn for all she taught and gave me and believe she knows how much she helped me. ∎

Ann Robinette, MS, RN, CS
1990

ELLIE

As the psychiatric nurse in a regional burn center, I provided crisis counseling to patients and families. Another part of my job was to help the nursing staff cope with the difficult emotional aspects of their jobs. Hope for a patient's future can be difficult to maintain when a patient sustains a severely disfiguring injury.

It had been a difficult summer. Our census had been high and many patients had died after prolonged efforts to save them. Staff was angry and discouraged. Jane was a 20-year-old college student who was severely burned in a car crash. She had 3rd-degree burns on her face, arms, and legs. Her face was destroyed and both of her arms required amputation. Plastic surgery could never restore even a likeness of her former face. Because her face was heavily bandaged and she was intubated she could not communicate with the staff. She became the girl without a face. Staff dreaded having to care for her.

Jane's widowed mother Ellie had come from her retirement home in Florida after the accident. She had no family or friends in the area. She had experienced tragedy in the past and believed that her faith would carry her and Jane through this adversity. Ellie could see Jane's amputations but it was impossible to convey to her the damage done to her daughter's face. She continued to express hope that at least her daughter's face could be restored through plastic surgery. I had always been an optimist about patients' futures. I had known other patients with severely disfiguring injuries who had built successful, fulfilling lives. I had not encountered injuries as severe as Jane's. I found it very difficult to communicate a sense of hope to Ellie about Jane's future. After the initial grafting, Jane had the bandages removed from her face. She remained intubated and still could not talk. Because of her swollen face, she could not even communicate with her eyes. Her mother and I had planned to go to Jane's room that afternoon so she could see her face before actually talking to her daughter for the first time without her bandages. As she looked through the window of Jane's room, horror crossed her face. She was unable to enter the room. When she returned to my office she was distraught and repulsed. She finally knew that her daughter's face could never be restored. She questioned why she had survived the accident. I could not find positive words to help her mother.

Ellie was staying at a local hotel. That evening she was in the nearly empty restaurant. A man sat at the table next to her. As they talked, she told the man about Jane's injuries and her sense of despair about her daughter's future. The man told her that he worked in the engineering department of the hospital. His son had died instantly in a car crash that summer. He became tearful and told Ellie, "If I could go to my son's grave and take him out, I would accept and treasure him no matter what was wrong with him. I would rather have my child on earth with me than dead." As the man left, he told her that he would stop by the Burn Center and see Ellie.

When I met with her the next day, she related the story to me. She described a sense of calm and acceptance that had overcome her because of this encounter. When the man did not visit, I helped Ellie contact the engineering department. She asked for the man by name. No one by that name worked there. She described him. The man was not in that department. We never did find the man, and she never saw him again.

There are times when there is no medicine to give or words to say to protect people from incredible pain. We all need that 'stranger' to remind us that our presence alone is a powerful source of recovery. ∎

Patricia Reddish, MSN, RN, CS
1985

TRAVIS

I was a staff nurse on an acute psychiatric unit. My days were filled with group therapies for orientation, education, and insight; individual relationship-building; and care of persons who did not or could not care for themselves. Some patients were very out of touch with my reality, others sad and despondent. Some were filled with energy that could make you dizzy.

Travis was in his mid 20s, suffered from schizophrenia, and had spent most of the previous year in the hospital. Travis had not been in the hospital continuously but had come in and out in a series of admissions. He would be admitted and the staff would cajole, coerce, bribe, and battle with Travis to take care of himself. He didn't want to take medicine. Travis rarely came to the group therapies offered and when he did attend (with much pushing), did not participate. And Travis would not bathe. About every 4th day we would do what was referred to as a 'show of force'—four or five staff escorted Travis to the shower—to insure that Travis showered. He wouldn't bathe or even wash up otherwise.

One morning I just could not face a battle with Travis over a

shower. This seemed so futile and not what I thought a nurse should do. Exasperated, I went into the wardroom where Travis slept, or at least stayed with the blanket pulled over his head. I plopped down on the foot of his bed and asked Travis to talk with me. With some patience and a few requests, he uncovered his head. I asked him why he came to the hospital when it appeared to me that he considered our requests and activities to be torture. He said it was the only place he had a friend, where anyone knew him or cared about him. I asked him if learning how to make friends might be a goal for this hospitalization and he was excited about this. We took a trip to the day room, Travis in his pj's, with greasy stringy hair and no slippers. I looked for the dirtiest patient in the day room and instructed Travis to try and talk with him. Travis went and sat next to the gentleman for about 30 seconds. He came running back to me. "I can't talk with him—he smells" Travis informed me. I asked him why the man smelled, and why couldn't he talk with him in spite of the odor? Travis took a shower that day without a 'show of force,' and, in fact, we never had to coerce a shower again.

Travis taught me to ask patients what they want, to move away from the same old methods, to try something new, and to trust the relationship to find the answers. I like to think Travis had a better life because we stopped struggling— I know I have.　　■

Ann Kelly, MSN, RN, CS
1978

THE RESIDENTS OF WARD 5

The enormous skeleton keys hanging from the waist of my fellow student nurses jangled as they lined up for lunch in our campus cafeteria. I was dreading my turn at our psychiatric rotation because I had heard very scary things about state hospital patients, and I knew I wasn't going to like it.

The first day on the locked ward confirmed my fears. As I walked slowly down the dark hall, I saw a disheveled lanky man heading straight toward me. "I'm from Mars...I'll let you ride in my spaceship if you like." That was enough for me. I headed into the dayroom, a smoke-filled hodgepodge of men, dressed in a variety of ill-fitting shirts and pants, who were either sitting in the ugly khaki-colored overstuffed chairs (most with cigarette burns in the upholstery) or pacing endlessly around trying to avoid each other's space. It was the same on the women's side, except that they were noisier (more high-pitched tones and emotional outbursts). One young woman dressed in a nightgown stood partially in the doorway of the dayroom. She stayed there for hours, drooling from the mouth, staring, swaying back and forth. I later found out this was Mary Jane's patient, and she was catatonic.

We were able to choose our patients, one from each side of the ward. Arlene was my female patient. She wasn't as scary as some, but most of the time what she said made no sense at all, so I mostly sat with her and listened. My professor said it was the nonverbal communication that really was important with these patients, since this was the only way we might have a chance of communicating and understanding one another. At first, I don't think she even knew I was there. She would talk into the air, ignoring me. It was uncomfortable to sit with her, because as a student nurse, I was used to being very busy and "doing" for patients. I felt as if I was wasting time, and I certainly couldn't be making a difference in Arlene's life, although it was comforting to know that no matter what I said I probably couldn't make her worse.

Paul was different. He didn't really seem 'crazy,' and he certainly didn't belong on this locked ward. His father was a psychiatrist, so that made it even more puzzling. Paul, just a few years younger than me, made sense when he talked and raced up and down the hallways talking to all the other patients. Paul came up to me the first day, so I thought it would be easy to work with him. He told me about his family, and we listened to his radio.

He often sang the words to "Nowhere Man," and I came to understand that 'isolation' was very real for him. Then one week he started running from me, hiding in the men's bathroom and shouting at me to go away. My professor suggested that I must be making an impact on him or he wouldn't be trying so hard to escape. I was upset. Being 'therapeutic' didn't feel good. I remember crying in some of my supervision sessions. It took awhile for me to understand that psychiatric nursing meant using who I was and expressing what I felt to help the patient deal with his emotions. This made me vulnerable, as Paul had made me cry, but if I could hang in there maybe Paul would realize that having someone who cared enough to listen to him was a positive interpersonal experience that he could tolerate and maybe enjoy.

That happened for both Paul and Arlene. Arlene had been writing nonsensical sentences and giving them to me during the last few weeks of my sitting with her. It seemed that she was trying to tell me something, but it was the schizophrenic's very personal language. The last day I spent with her I found her in her usual dayroom chair, but she was dressed neatly, had put her makeup on with appropriate restraint and subtlety, and she actually looked pretty. "I have a present for you." She handed me a note. It was one of her nature pictures that she drew, a simple childlike yellow crayon of the sun. There was the familiar unintelligible mixture of partial sentences and word salad, but in among this was "I missed you." What a gift to give me! She had actually managed to not only dress appropriately, a nonverbal message to acknowledge our relationship, but she had communicated verbally as well!

Paul started talking to me again the day I observed him in his insulin coma treatment and was with him when he woke up. He was really a captive audience—the recovery room allowed no means of escape from me. The week before I left, he suggested we could go to church together. My professor helped me understand that he was asking me for a date but had made it sound more acceptable since he knew I went to a Lutheran college. The last day with Paul was spent with me declining our 'date' but telling him what talking to him had meant to me. "Well," he said, "even though we're not going to church together, I guess we had a 'groovy kind of love.'" That was just like Paul to borrow words from a song to tell me how he felt. ∎

Margo Foltz Wilson, MS, RN, CS, CGP
1966

JANE

When I first started working in this very busy ICU (it was the biggest military hospital in the United States), I felt frightened and overwhelmed by the vast spectrum of patients. There were many young patients: motor vehicle accidents, traumas, gunshot wounds, and very aggressive cancers. We also took care of surgical patients after open-heart surgery, neurosurgery, and many other potentially life-threatening surgeries.

One day, I was assigned 'the code bed.' This is a bed saved for any life-threatening emergency that occurs within the hospital. These beds were almost always filled before the close of the shift. Also assigned to the code bed with me was my mentor, Mary. Mary was a wonderful nurse. As a new nurse to the unit, I had watched her and was impressed by her compassion and expertise. Patients under Mary's care invariably did well. I chose Mary as my role model and she reveled in the task.

As we performed the checks we do while awaiting an assignment, a 'code blue' was called over the overhead paging system. We knew that if this person survived the code blue, he or she would be our patient. Our hearts sank as we heard that the location of the code was the obstetrics suite. Obstetric

emergencies were rare but usually severe. A woman's uterus or womb is such a vascular organ that she can literally bleed to death before interventions by the medical team can be of help. We were notified that the woman in question had been rushed to surgery and shortly thereafter a second code blue was called from the operating room.

Amazingly, the mother survived and was brought to the ICU from surgery accompanied by an entourage of surgeons, obstetricians, and anesthesiologists. She was our patient. Jane was intubated and connected to a respirator that would support her breathing. She had undergone a cesarean section and had given birth to a healthy baby boy, her third child. Unknown to the obstetricians performing Jane's cesarean was the fact that Jane had placenta accreta, a rare condition in which the placenta invades the musculature of the uterus. When the baby and the placenta were removed, Jane hemorrhaged.

Jane's care was complex and demanding. She had had an emergency hysterectomy in surgery and we continued to transfuse her with massive amounts of blood products, several units at a time. Our first problem was that Jane was not stabilizing. Her belly, which was distended and full of blood, was getting bigger. Her heart rate, which was running at twice its normal rate, was getting faster. "She's still bleeding from somewhere" Mary said, and I knew she was right. Jane went to surgery a second time.

Jane's stay in the ICU was long. Her husband, the captain of a Navy ship, was called home. He was told on three separate occasions that Jane would die. Mary and I were her primary nurses. We played 'tag team' nursing with Jane: if Mary had a day off, I took care of Jane and vice versa. Some days Jane was so sick and her care was so intense that it took both of us to provide the care she needed. We were determined that Jane was not going to die.

Jane succumbed to all the complications of severe hypovolemic shock. Her kidneys failed, she went through a course of dialysis, and finally her renal function returned. Her lungs became stiff and it became difficult for her to get enough oxygen, and once again we thought we were going to lose her. Because Jane had been on the ventilator for a long time, it was necessary for her to have a tracheotomy performed. Jane developed a GI bleed, as a result of the stress her body had been under. She was rushed back to the operating room for a subtotal gastrectomy, and a portion of her stomach was removed.

It became difficult to keep Jane's spirits up in her day-to-day care. As soon as one system healed another would fail. Although Jane was a fighter, I could sense the futility that had engulfed her as she spent day after day going through often painful procedures and never seeing the outside of that hospital room. Finally, I walked into my next day taking care of Jane with ammunition.

As I suctioned Jane's trach, I talked to her about being at home and sitting in her favorite chair in her favorite sunny room watching her boys play. I asked her to imagine that she was there and not in the ICU. I found out that Jane loved chocolate, and so we would discuss chocolate in its many forms.

Jane eventually recovered and was discharged. Life in the ICU went on. Months went by and there were always more very sick patients.

One day I was busy with a patient when I noticed Jane's dad in my peripheral vision. He had someone with him, someone I didn't recognize. He was carrying a box. He approached me gingerly and questioned, "Hazel?" I looked up and the person with him stared at me. She was very thin, and as I looked at her I noticed the scar on her neck that had been left by a tracheotomy. All at once it clicked. "Jane!" I said as the tears poured down both of our cheeks. "I brought some chocolate eclairs" she said, as we hugged. ■

Hazel M. Harrison, RN, CCRN
1990

DAWN

When I met Dawn, I was working as a nurse practitioner in a clinic that served all medical assistance patients. Dawn was sitting on the exam table holding an infant at her breast. Four other children sat on the floor. Dawn was such a beautiful young woman with smooth, clear black skin. And she was crying. The tears gave a glistening to her makeup. I said simply, "Dawn, what is wrong?" She reached into the pockets of her jeans and pulled out a piece of paper containing her GED results. She cried, "I can't do math."

She told me the story of her troubled and abusive childhood in Texas. She wanted to continue her schooling to make a better life for her family. We talked a little about the GED and about some ways to study, and finally, took care of the sore throat she had come in for.

A few months later she came to the clinic again. She said that she was having anxiety attacks. Indicating the paper she had pulled from her jeans, Dawn said that she had failed the math section again. I thought for a moment and then asked her, "Do you know how to shoot craps?" She looked at me strangely. "Yes," she replied with some reservation. "Why?" I asked her to tell me what she did when she played the game. She replied slowly, "Throw the dice." After a moment's hesitation, she continued, talking about quickly adding the numbers so she would not be cheated. Then she described counting the number of throws to determine the chances of her winning. Delighted, I replied, "Then you can do math! You're already doing it, and probability too." She responded first with incredulity and then with a growing excitement. We discussed how to put this together to pass the test.

In late May, a smiling, happy Dawn brought me an invitation to her graduation ceremony. She would be marching with the local high school to get her GED. Thanks to a little patience and a lot of "crap." ∎

Joyce Knestrick, PhD(C), FNP,
RN
1996

31

MR. JONES

I am a post anesthesia care unit nurse and have helped thousands of patients move from a deep anesthetized sleep to 'awake and stable.' Unfortunately, few of my patients ever know I am even there, let alone what part I play in their safe recovery. Thankless to some, maybe, but it has given me the unique opportunity to experience a side of human nature rarely seen.

In one such memory, late in my shift, I received Mr. Jones. Although he had undergone a simple surgery, an endotracheal tube, maintaining his airway until he was alert enough to breathe on his own, remained in place. He was otherwise stable and just needed to let the anesthesia wear off and wake up. Unfortunately, minutes later I received a second patient, Mr. Bates, who was not okay. He woke up from his appendectomy, then his neck started to swell. He was having a great deal of difficulty breathing and was becoming more anxious by the minute. Doctors, nurses, and technicians crowded around the bedside. Meanwhile, Mr. Jones soundly slept on, with just a hospital curtain separating him from all the excitement. Physician consults, lab tests, respiratory treatments, and a multitude of IV drugs were given to Mr. Bates before the swelling went down. His neck returned to its normal size and he could once again breathe easily.

Another nurse had stepped in to monitor Mr. Jones, who was still asleep and oblivious to the critical situation that had taken place, less than a foot from where he lay. As I resumed his care, I touched his shoulder and said "Mr. Jones, wake up, your surgery is over." He opened his eyes. I removed his airway tube and he immediately said, "You know, I don't feel well, call 911 for me." ■

Christine Rodighiero, RN
1995

MR. ARNOLD

As I passed Mr. Arnold's room on the medical ward, I heard the urgent-sounding intonation of his nurse's voice: "Somebody, I need help in here." I entered the room to find Mr. Arnold clenching his chest, as he stated "This is the worst pain I have ever had."

I was aware that Mr. Arnold was scheduled for a balloon angioplasty later that day. My instincts told me that he was having a heart attack and needed to have his right coronary artery opened up immediately, so that blood could flow through it to nourish the heart muscle. I immediately took an electrocardiogram and noted the ominous signs of impending heart attack. I called the patient's cardiologist and arranged for Mr. Arnold to be taken to the catheterization laboratory to undergo the angioplasty procedure, accompanied by several student nurses, who were eager to learn all about Mr. Arnold's urgent situation. I mentored them in understanding the architecture of his coronary arteries, how the angioplasty procedure worked, and how to read the abnormal changes on his electrocardiogram.

Soon after the procedure began, Mr. Arnold's blood pressure dropped dangerously low. He needed emergency measures, including an intraaortic balloon pump. This device was inserted into the large femoral artery in his groin and positioned in his aorta. The end of the catheter was connected to a pump to push helium into the balloon within the aorta, which then pushed the blood out ahead of the heart's contraction. This device made the heart's own pumping action easier.

Suddenly the scene escalated into a whirlwind of activity. Simultaneously I focused on my responsibility to the student nurses—to teach and afford them a good learning experience. Suddenly, one of the nurses exclaimed "His oxygen saturation is dropping." Mr. Arnold was no longer able to sustain breathing on his own. Preparations were made to place a tube in his windpipe and connect him to a ventilator.

The respiratory therapist, who was at the head of the table, suddenly turned to me and said "He's saying 'nurse'." As I approached Mr. Arnold, he held out his pale, clammy hand and managed a weak squeeze as I placed my hand in his. In a soft, fading voice, he whispered "Judy, please let me see Judy." Mr. Arnold was a widower and his only daughter lived out of state. Suddenly, I saw the picture with great clarity. From his point of view, his most immediate need was to be able to speak to his daughter.

The cardiologist commanded, "Get him intubated now." The respiratory therapist nudged me out of the way to prepare to place the tube into Mr. Arnold's throat. Mr. Arnold's oxygen level was dropping but was not yet to the critical level. I believed that there was time to honor his request. I leaned over to Mr. Arnold, stroked his forehead, and reassured him that I would try to call Judy, so that he could hear her voice. Luckily, Judy answered on the third ring. I placed the portable phone beside his ear. He told his daughter that he loved her, and thereafter, a breathing tube was placed.

It was 'touch and go' for awhile, but the angioplasty procedure was successful and Mr. Arnold made a full recovery. Approximately 6 months later, I received a page. It was from the hospital information desk. The volunteer explained, "Two people are here and insist on seeing you." It was Mr. Arnold and his daughter. They thanked me for giving them that moment. They revealed their then unexpressed fear that Mr. Arnold would not survive. They both were most grateful for the medical expertise that had saved his life, but they wanted me to know that my making it possible for them to connect by phone was, at that moment, the most important moment in their lives. They asked me never to forget what it meant to them and made me promise that if I were ever in that situation again, I would remember how important it is for a critically ill patient to feel the security of a family member's love and support.

I am proud of my scientific cardiovascular nursing knowledge, but realize that it pales in comparison to being able to relate to the patient's needs and put them first, especially at a very critical moment. It was a valuable lesson learned and I am a better nurse and person for this experience. ∎

Susan Quaal, PhD, APRN, CVS, CCRN
1992

THE HOLIDAY GRIEF GROUP

In December I was asked to make a presentation at the local hospice on grief and the holidays, to help families who had lost loved ones share and talk about the hardship. The hospice had never sponsored one of these programs before but they thought there was a real need. Often people who were grieving felt isolated and alone, especially during the holidays.

As a clinical nurse specialist in private practice, I had often been asked to run groups focusing on wellness and stress reduction. This kind of group was a little different, and I wanted to provide an atmosphere where people felt safe enough to share their feelings.

As the time approached for the group, the hospice director told me that only a few people had signed up. I was disappointed but we decided to go ahead with it anyway, feeling that even if there were only a small group, those there could benefit from the sharing. When I arrived, however, there were already 12 people in the

Mary Anne La Torre, MA, RN, CCNS
1997

room and they continued to come in until we had about 18. I felt overwhelmed momentarily with the unexpected size and response.

As we went around the room, family members introduced themselves and talked a little about the death of their loved one. When we got to Sarah, she began to cry and then apologized profusely for doing so. She explained that her family didn't like to see her cry, and so she held back, believing it would make everyone uncomfortable. Many of the members of the group reassured her that this was not so and that she had a right to cry. I said "It's important to give yourself permission to feel and grieve as you need to—not as anybody else wants you to." This made her cry more as she described how stressful the holidays were. She was going to be taking care of her mother and children while trying to maintain a calmness she did not feel. Sarah's crying seemed to touch us all. Members shared their own pain. Some cried along with her and everyone encouraged her to be herself rather than pretending she felt something else. In the process, as members encouraged her, they gave themselves permission as well.

When we ended and broke for coffee, the group members continued to share with each other, many coming up and hugging Sarah and each other. I felt blessed to be a part of the group. When she left, Sarah gave me a hug and said "Whatever happens, I feel I can make it through the holidays now." It was a Christmas gift I will remember. ∎

BLANCA

The phone rang early on a Sunday evening. It was the unit. There had been several ICU patients admitted and they had a staffing problem. They asked if I would I come in to work on night shift. Something told me to say "yes." It was more than the typical guilt response, but I didn't know what. I was the head nurse and I hadn't been needed on the off shifts very much.

The shift started out normally and I was assigned two patients. One of my patients was an 18-year-old Hispanic burn patient. Her name was Blanca and she had extensive injuries. In intensive care, the crisis environment is a barrier to interpersonal interaction between patients and nurses. Therefore, we really knew very little about her, and the focus had been on her physical care to save her life.

At night, a part of the patient care plan is to try to provide for some rest, even in critical care. In the middle of the night after completing Blanca's treatments, I asked her where her home was. She started to talk and I sat down in the chair beside her. She told me about her life as a migrant farm worker and the crops she liked to pick the most.

They worked the seasonal crops and she had been what sounded like everywhere. She liked Michigan and the cherry season the best. She talked about her home in south Texas and how much she missed it. Many families are U.S. citizens and live in the Valley and work as migrant workers up North. She wanted to know whether I knew that. I said I did and shared with her that my family had just moved to McAllen, Texas. It was very close to her home. I reached out to hold her hand, and then she said, "No one has bothered to care about me or wanted to know about me." She talked about the accident. "It couldn't have been prevented." It happened in the migrant housing where she and her family were living and working. She talked about how hard it was being one of the oldest and having to do the migrant work and help with the other children, but yet she missed all of them. They had left Colorado for the next crop and would be back in a month. She needed to rest, and then I knew that this must have been why I was guided to say "yes, I will work tonight."

A human connection was created between Blanca and myself. Her surprise at my 'caring' about her and taking the time to listen helped her to know that her life was important. Listening, an act of caring, created a connection and acceptance. Working that night shift gave me more than Blanca—a lived experience of the significance of the simple act of listening and gift of acceptance that comes with it. ∎

Mickey L. Parsons, PhD, RN
1973

SETH

It seemed like such a simple problem to resolve, but Seth could find no answers or relief. He was young and had been so full of life. The sky had been the limit. He was now experiencing pelvic pain that prevented him from working, attending school, and satisfying his wife. The pain had started in earnest 5 years ago when he was 24 years old. At 29, the pain was ruining his life.

Seth had been to every type of physician imaginable and had still not found relief. As a last measure, he was referred to me in hopes that behavioral therapy could assist him in identifying and eliminating his pain.

I had recently attended a nursing conference where I heard a nurse speak on the benefits of using behavioral techniques to eliminate pelvic pain in females. However, I knew little about how these techniques could assist males. I had intended to return to my job and see if there was an area where these techniques could be used. Little did I know that I would have a referral so soon.

On our first meeting, I could tell that Seth was weary from the pain that was now controlling his life. He was a tall, African American male, who entered the room with his head lowered and shoulders slumped.

After a brief conversation, it was apparent that Seth was motivated to do whatever necessary to restore his life. I made no promises nor did I tell him that I had never tried this therapy before. I wanted him to be optimistic and to have hope.

Belief in the ability to control one's body can be a powerful motivating agent. People no longer feel like victims but feel the power of their inner will to change the way their body is functioning.

We then identified trigger points that initiated Seth's pain. This was done simply with an applicator stick and slight pressure. Then I used cold and heat to anesthetize, relax, and soothe the muscles that were causing him burning, pelvic pain. Biofeedback assisted him with visually understanding what he was doing with his pelvic floor muscles and how it felt when they were relaxed. Through sensation, he was able to identify when he was tensing his pelvic floor muscles. In addition, we examined foods that may have been intensifying his pain and worked to eliminate them from his diet.

Seth was elated. He realized that he had been tensing his pelvic floor muscles and was totally unaware. He was ready to go home and practice the muscle relaxation regimen on a daily basis and willingly restrict his diet. I advised him not to overdo his new assignment.

He returned the following week a believer. The pain was subsiding. In fact, he had brief periods of relief that he had not experienced in years. I reinforced the fact that he would have to continue this relaxation regimen for the rest of his life, sometimes more intensely than others. We all experience stress, and some of us carry it in our neck muscles, some in our stomachs, some in our bowel, and others in our pelvic floor musculature area. The importance is knowing how your stress expresses itself and spending time each day to relieve it.

After 4 weeks of therapy, Seth's pain was gone. He was ecstatic to be pain free. He walked in the room for his last visit, head held high, standing tall.

"I want to thank you" he said. "Now I can begin to live my life again."

I was so excited that he had such a remarkable recovery. However, I felt it very important to leave him with the thought that his success was the product of his efforts. "You did it" I said. "You are the one that made the program work."

"Thanks, Teach. I will make you proud" he replied.

These words continue to ring in my ears when I have a patient who is challenging and resisting therapy. We gave each other the gift of knowing that the body can learn and relearn with gentle coaxing, attention, and caring. ∎

Angela C. Joseph, MSN, RN, CURN
1993

MICHELLE

I was working as a transplant coordinator at a university system when I met Michelle. She was a 16-year-old Hispanic girl who had undergone a right lung transplant for primary pulmonary hypertension approximately 2 years ago.

Michelle had returned to school and was very active in taking care of her little brother. Both her parents worked and had a poor understanding of her illness. Unfortunately, Michelle had started experiencing signs and symptoms of chronic rejection. She was not a candidate for retransplantation, so her options were limited. We tried changing her antirejection medications but were unsuccessful. Approximately 6 months after I met Michelle, it became clear to everyone that she would not live much longer.

Our team met with Michelle to explain that she would not be retransplanted and would likely die soon. Michelle accepted the news with grace and calmness. Her first statement was " Who will take care of my little brother?" Her parents were devastated and did not understand what was happening. Michelle explained to them that her lungs were not working and could

Kate Morse, MS, RN, ANP-C,
ACNP, CCRN
1996

not be fixed this time. She wanted to go home, think about things, and come back to the clinic the following week. I checked in with her at home and she continued to amaze me with her questions about death and dying. She told me she was not afraid to die but was worried about what her family would do without her.

She was readmitted about 10 days later with further heart problems. I sat on her bed and asked her if she had any questions about dying. She told me that she had picked out the dress she would wear at her funeral and the music she wanted played. Again, she told me very calmly that she was not afraid to die, but worried about who would play with her little brother and was sad that she would not be able to go to college. She had wanted to be a pharmacist. We discharged her home with hospice care and weren't sure if we would see her again.

About a week later Michelle called me to tell me about a dream she had. She dreamt that the doorbell rang and when she answered it her lung donor was there and told her that it was time to give back her lung. Michelle felt strongly that she would die very soon and wanted to say thank-you. Her mother called me 2 days later and said that Michelle had died at home in her sleep.

I will never forget the courage and grace that Michelle displayed facing her own death at such a young age. She helped me as a nurse to see that death is a natural part of living and that we all move in and out of the circle of life. ∎

CLYDE

The call from surgery telling me my next patient was on his way up came around 10 pm. When I asked for details about the patient, I was told he was a male in his early 30s who had attempted a jail break that afternoon. He had jumped out of an 8th-story window to gain his freedom. What he had gotten was a fractured pelvis and both legs shattered. He had been in surgery for hours and was coming to the recovery room in a full body plaster cast from his chin to his toes.

A few minutes later, Clyde rolled in. He was indeed in a full body cast and because he was a fugitive, his leg, in the cast, was handcuffed to the bed. At the time I remember thinking how absurd this seemed. The man was barely conscious, and with his cast he certainly wasn't going anywhere! After checking him in and giving me the report of how the surgery had proceeded, the operating nurses left me, to go back downstairs. I was left alone with my patient. I jumped into action, taking his vital signs, asking him if he was in any pain, and trying to make him comfortable while he breathed off the anesthesia, and so I was surprised to hear a noise at the door. At first it sounded like a tentative knock, which I ignored. No visitors were allowed in the recovery room.

The next thing I knew a man was standing beside me with a gun pointed at my face. He looked more frightened than I felt. I stood there wondering which drugs this man wanted to steal. My mind was racing with the thought that I had not been taught how to deal with a robber, and I was indignant that this man was in "my" recovery room. I did not want to get hurt, and I was not stupid. I was prepared to give him whatever he wanted to take, except the one thing I was amazed he requested.

He looked around to be sure we were alone and then he demanded that I hand over Clyde! He told me he had come to break Clyde out and finish the job that Clyde had attempted that afternoon. I could not believe my ears. This man was going to kidnap my unconscious patient! I calmly told him that his friend was in a full body cast and was handcuffed to the bed. The man came to the bedside to examine Clyde. Clyde was not awake enough to acknowledge his rescuer, and I told the man that he was more than welcome to take Clyde and the bed, which he was going to need to transport Clyde. I even volunteered to help disconnect Clyde from the monitors and push him out the door to the elevators for the ride to the first floor and the door to "freedom."

As soon as the door to the elevator closed, I walked back into the recovery room and called the policeman who was sitting at his usual station at the entrance to the hospital. I informed him that a man had just robbed me at gunpoint and had taken my most precious possession at that moment, my patient. I told him the patient was stable, barely conscious, in a full body cast, and handcuffed to the bed. I also stated that his friend was obviously stupid, unstable, armed, and headed his way.

Thirty long minutes later, my patient was returned to me. He was now awake, in pain, and visibly upset. His friend was on his way to jail. The police officer assured me he would be staying with me in the recovery room and Clyde would have a full time guard until he was returned to jail. Many hospital policies were created as a result of this incident. ∎

Renee P. McLeod MSN, RN, CPNP
1976

KEN

At 9:30 pm on a Sunday night, I was working on a coronary step-down unit. Mr. Dudek's family had just left. Ken Dudek, a 60-year-old man, had been hospitalized with a heart attack. His cardiologist had performed a heart catheterization on Friday to assess the damage to his heart. The cardiologist was recommending open-heart surgery to hopefully prevent any future heart attacks.

Mr. Dudek had agreed to surgery, scheduled for Monday morning. I had been waiting for his visitors to leave so that I could begin the skin preparation for surgery. The skin prep consisted of the patient showering and then scrubbing himself with a scrub brush, filled with an antiseptic that would remain on his skin overnight. I had explained the procedure to Mr. Dudek earlier in the shift. Still, I got the sense that he wasn't anxious to get started.

"Did you have a nice visit with your family?" I asked.

"Yes, but we are all a little nervous" Mr. Dudek replied.

"Rightfully so. You've been through a very major event. It must have been frightening" I stated.

"You know though, Marlys, after the pain stopped and I saw

my wife's face and knew I was still alive, I wasn't frightened anymore. What is troubling me now is all the things in my life that I wished I had done more of or differently."

I was all of 21 years old at the time and probably didn't grasp the complexity of the reflection, but nonetheless I asked him "What would you have done differently?"

His response, "I would have taken my wife to Alaska. Alaska is the most beautiful place I've ever seen. When I was young, I traveled to many places, but Alaska has always had my heart. I've told my wife about the incredible mountains and the open space and told her that sometime soon we would visit it together. But somehow the time was never right. Now we finally have the money to travel and this has to happen."

"Do you think that because you have had heart problems that you won't be able to travel?" I asked.

"Do you think I can still go?"

"You'd have to clear it with your physician, but with proper preparation you should be able to show your bride Alaska!"

"No kidding? Well, let's get this show on the road then! The sooner it's over, the sooner we can start making our plans."

Six months later I received a postcard from Alaska. The note read "Thanks for taking the time to listen and reassure me that my life wasn't over. Alaska is just as beautiful as I remember it. My wife and I are having a great time. Ken Dudek."

∎

Marlys Vespe, MSN, RN
1978

ROSIE

As a patient advocate, I listen to many patients and family members talk to me about their concerns.

Expecting Rosie, I was surprised to see Rosie, her three children (all adults), and their pastor. As we sat in the small conference room, each member talked of their memories of Keith as a father, a husband, a friend. Many tears were shed as they each talked about him.

We talked about his hospitalization. Keith had many health problems. He was legally blind, diabetic with foot sores, and had numerous heart problems and neurological difficulties. Rosie didn't feel he was treated as an individual with unique needs while a patient in our hospital. She needed to share this since she was stuck in her grieving and couldn't seem to move on. She wanted to tell us so we would learn from Keith's experience and make it better for the next patient. I told her we were committed to sticking by her, so her story would be heard and we would walk with her through her feelings until she felt some resolution. Tears flowed, both from the family and me as they shared their grief.

This meeting led to meetings with nurses from the stations Keith was on and meetings with the nurse practice board, as we listened to Rosie tell her story. She wanted nurses in the hospital to know more about Keith and, hopefully, to learn what had been important to both of them. She relayed her story of the devoted wife of a man suffering from chronic illnesses. I wasn't sure if putting her through the telling of her story over and over again would, in the end, help her in her grief process or just torment her. I let her take the lead in calling me when she felt the need.

After several months, the meetings became less frequent and I stopped getting calls from Rosie. I thought about her many times and wondered how she was doing. It wasn't until months later that I had my answer. Around mid-December, a card was delivered to my office. On the outside it said "Peace." Inside it said "Couldn't get through the holidays without wishing you much happiness and to thank you again for your kindness!" Tears welled up as I stared at the card. I knew Rosie was all right and would continue on her journey. ∎

Rose Weintraub, RN
1987

ALICE

"Oh no, I wish I weren't starting my psych rotation." My thoughts were racing as I entered the large conference area for orientation. "I never know what to say when someone is hurting emotionally." A group of 18 student nurses had gathered to learn our specific assignments for the next 3 months.

"Miss Warner, you will be assigned Miss Alice Ferguson in C-632. She has been with us for over 10 years and to our knowledge, she has never communicated verbally with anyone."

"She is not violent, she just sits there all day long, day after day. Because you love to talk so much, maybe she will respond to you." As I approached C-632, I looked inside and saw a woman sitting in a well-worn arm chair, facing the window. I entered the room and called Miss Ferguson's name. There was no sign of recognition or acknowledgement. I spoke again—still no response. Knowing I would have to report back on my first visit, I decided to approach my patient at a closer range. "Miss Ferguson, my name is Miss Warner, and I will be your nurse each day for the next 3 months. May I sit down?" There was still no response, only a brief glance that acknowledged she heard me. I sat there for about 5 minutes, very quiet, not moving. It

came to me very gently and very quietly to just spend each day sitting by her side, and not saying a word, just being present. I remained obedient to that nudge, until it was time to leave. As I stood up ready to go I said "Miss Ferguson, I am leaving now, but I will be back to spend time with you tomorrow." Her response was a brief nod of her head.

During the next week, each day I would introduce my arrival, acknowledge her presence, pull up a chair and quietly sit beside her, until it was time for me to leave. At that time I would speak of my departure and remind her of my return the next day.

Each day the silence became easier to endure. During my second week, in addition to announcing my arrival, I informed Miss Ferguson that I would be with her each day, at the same designated time, and that my visits would continue for 10½ more weeks. I also let her know that I would be open to anything she wanted to say or chose not to say, but that I would be there every day no matter what.

The weeks passed: week 2, week 3, week 4. Nothing seemed to change. Then on Monday of the 5th week, I noticed that Alice had pulled my chair a little closer to her, with it actually facing her. I inquired if she desired me to sit in the chair as it was placed and she again nodded slightly. "Thank you for being open to our visits, I do enjoy my time with you, and I will continue to be here as promised each day." I was surprised to actually hear myself stating that I enjoyed the silence, me, who grew up being called "the mouth."

At the conclusion of the 5th week, without lifting her head, Alice said "thank you." I said good-bye, walked outside and began to cry. Alice had actually spoken to me. "How exciting," I thought, "I wonder what will happen during the remaining 7 weeks."

The following week Alice began to greet me with "good morning" and my departure with "good-bye," but still we spoke nothing in between. We were both feeling increasingly comfortable with our silence, and occasionally I would add a slight statement about how important my time was with her, or comment briefly about how she looked or what I saw outside the window.

One day during the 9th week, Alice looked at me directly and asked "Why do you stay with me each day?" I felt my hands tighten around the arm of the chair in surprise, and with an even voice responded "Because I enjoy being with you and feel comfortable in this room." Alice looked at me again, and said "No one has ever done this before, they always leave. Thank you for staying with me." I felt my eyes begin to water. Alice responded with a smile, a beautiful smile, and I noticed she too had tears in her eyes.

"I will be with you for 3 more weeks and then my rotation is over, but I will be here each day during that time." I felt I had to be honest with her, because I knew that Alice should be aware of my remaining days with her. The next day when I arrived, I noticed Alice had put on some lipstick and pulled her hair back with a soft pink ribbon. She was lovely. I wanted to embrace her but did so mentally in respect of her privacy. "Oh Miss Ferguson, you look so lovely today, this is a special day." The words just slipped out, but Alice nodded and said "Yes it is. You see, today is my 63rd birthday and I have never spent my birthday with anyone since I was 33 years old." I wanted to jump up and hug Alice, but I knew I couldn't, so I gently commented on how special it was for me as well. Alice reached out her hand and shook mine. "Thank you Miss Warner for being here with me, it means more than I can tell you." As I got up to leave Alice said "Tomorrow is a special day and I'll look forward to seeing you." We smiled and parted closer than I had ever felt possible. The next day I brought her a single pink rose and wished her a happy birthday. As Alice reached for her rose, she started sobbing and sat down with her face buried in her hands. "Oh Miss Warner, Miss Warner," she spoke between the sobs in a slow but deliberate manner. "I have never talked to anyone about this ever, but over the past weeks, I have grown to trust you, like I have never trusted anyone in my life."

Alice began to speak as if she needed to get everything out

immediately. "It was the day after my 32nd birthday. My boyfriend had asked me to marry him. I said yes, and it was the happiest day of my life. We needed to wait until he returned from overseas duty, which would be in 1 year. I agreed and we both felt a bond of love that we knew would last forever. Later on that evening before he left we had sex together. I knew it was wrong, but I loved him so much and I knew we would be together forever. He left the next morning. Two weeks later I received a message that he had been killed in a car accident. I was devastated and felt my world had come to an end. I couldn't talk to anyone and decided to keep my pain to myself. To make it even worse, I found out that I was pregnant. I was ashamed and embarrassed and was unable to tell anyone. I couldn't have the baby of a man who was dead, when I wasn't married. So I took a coat hanger and I caused my baby to abort, and I buried it outside my window." At this point Alice was sobbing uncontrollably. I felt I needed to reach out and hold her, and when I did she just clung to me and cried for a long, long time. I just held her, and quietly prayed for God's tenderness and healing presence to enfold her.

When she finally stopped crying, she told me that for 31 years she had held this inside her, for 31 years she had ached, and for 31 years she kept silent about her abortion and her entire life. In essence, she never spoke again to anyone, at any time, regarding anything. She had been institutionalized for the past 25 years, never sharing with anyone. "For the first time, I can trust someone. You were there for me every day and I knew you would be there for me no matter what." Alice left the hospital 2 weeks later, with the notation of a miraculous recovery. I knew that the real miracle had unfolded through the gift of listening, the blessing of trust, and the bond of sharing. ∎

Carmen Germaine Warner,
MSN, RN, FAAN
1962

MR. HUBNER

When I was a recent graduate, there was an elderly gentleman, Mr. Hubner, with lung cancer. He was dying. He knew it. . .his wife knew it. . . his grown children knew it. . . I knew it. . . his doctors knew it. Yet, everyday they'd come and take him for radiation treatment. But one day, when I was getting him ready to go, he told me he didn't want to go anymore. He said the table was hard. It was painful to be moved. He wanted to get cleaned up, shave, put on clean pajamas, and spend the day with his wife of so many years.

I told him he didn't have to go and refused to let the orderly take him. The radiologist called me. He was furious. He accused me of trying to kill the man. . .he said I was "taking away his only chance." I said he didn't want to go and he wasn't going. I gave the man a bath. I shaved him. I sat him up in bed and had his wife come in.

He died that afternoon and, while the doctors were pronouncing him dead, I sat in the solarium with his wife. She was an elderly, frail woman who had spent her entire adult life with this man. I sat down beside her, not saying a word. She took my hand and held it. She never said a word, either.

Since my days in training and my early years as a nurse, there have been so many patients, so many families, so many situations in hospitals and in outpatient settings, in medical and psychiatric nursing. Through all of the years, all of the patients have been important—but it was the early years that seem most important in establishing a foundation for all that lay ahead. I'm convinced that I, as a nurse, would never have been able to bear all I have had to bear without that foundation, and maybe even a calling.

It was during those early years that I learned from the nurses and patients who taught me, that I established who I was going to be as a nurse, and what was going to matter. Somewhere, somehow, I, like so many other nurses, decided that patients and moments were what mattered. I treasure every card, every note, and every memory of those early years—as well as every moment of all the years that have followed. ■

Kelly Gaul, MSN, RN, CS
1975

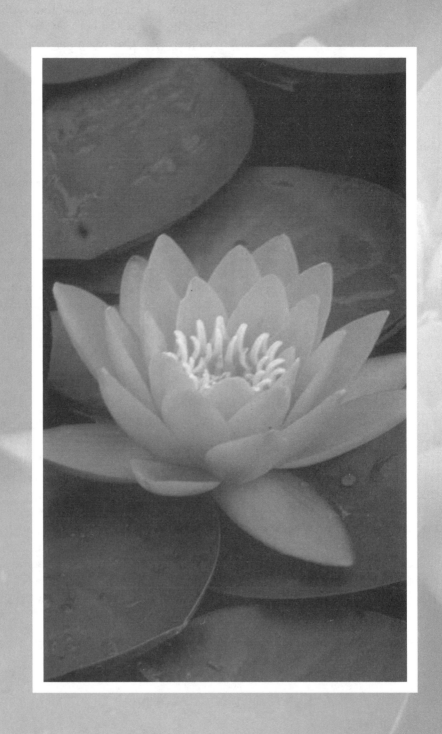

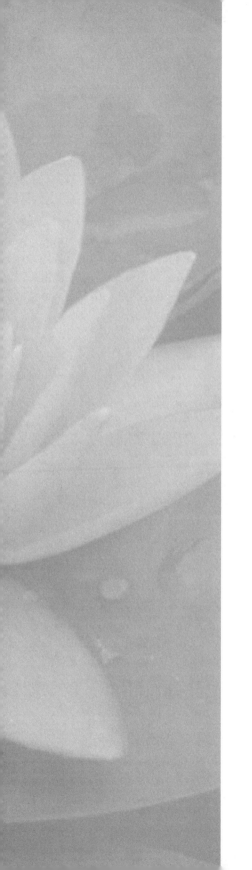

LOVE

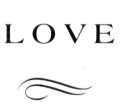

AMY

I had not been able to find a job as a pediatric nurse practitioner. Finally I saw an ad in the paper: a nurse midwife had opened her own practice in a rural area and was looking for a partner. I had a 3-year-old daughter and a 3-month-old son, and I was looking for a job where I could set my own hours and have some freedom from a 9-to-5 job.

It seemed like a match made in heaven. I would help Teri deliver babies, and then I would have babies to see in my growing practice! We worked out of the basement of a house where we provided prenatal care, childbirth and parenting classes, and in a corner I set up an office where I could see the newborn babies. Often patients paid by bartering for other services. For example, we had secretarial help for a year, and I had the basement of our house finished and painted by the father of a baby in my practice. I had planned to see all of the newborns during the day with my baby by my side, but I quickly realized that to bring some patients into my practice I had to attend the births.

I knew from the first time I met Laura that this birth would be different. This family had a "family bed," which was many beds pushed together. Everyone in the family,

which consisted of Laura and her husband and 4 children, who ranged in age from 2 to 8 years old, slept in this big bed. In the closet was another twin bed that Laura and her husband used when they wanted some privacy. Each time a baby was born a new bed was added.

When I arrived, Laura was in active labor. All of the children were cuddled in the bed with Laura while she worked hard to bring the newest member of the family into the world. I crawled onto the bed with everyone else and provided words of comfort and support as Teri attended Laura. Right before sunrise, Amy decided to be born. Laura's husband woke the sleeping children so everyone could watch. Teri put the newborn on Laura's abdomen and cut the cord. Laura promptly put the baby to her breast. While I quickly examined the baby to be sure she was fine, Laura's husband took off his shirt and had each of the children take off their tops. Laura then handed the newborn to her husband. I watched in awe as he cuddled the naked baby to his bare chest and had the children do the same. As he did so, he introduced each child to their new little sister. They warmed up the baby by providing skin-to-skin contact. It was the most incredible sight I have ever seen. After checking on Amy one more time, I thanked the family for letting me be a part of this beautiful birth. Teri and I closed the door and headed downstairs, where Laura's friends and family had prepared a celebration breakfast. I knew I had found the right job. ∎

Renee P. McLeod, MSN, RN, CPNP
1982

JOEY

During my years of working in a large urban teaching hospital's CICU, I had been called to the emergency department to help only on a few occasions. This was one of them. I chose Gail, a dear friend, and great critical care nurse colleague, to accompany me on this call for help.

It was the Fourth of July. We were told a severely injured male was en route from a fireworks explosion. Of course we immediately thought "some kids playing with fireworks." Just before his arrival we were told the male was only 14 years old. Before the days of regional trauma programs, cases like this were treated in an operating room within an emergency department—that is, if the ED was lucky enough to have one. The young patient arrived by stretcher and was treated in our ED/OR accompanied by a group of the hospital's best staff.

On first impression, he looked tan. Then we realized his skin was burned, mostly off. All of his hair, brows, and lashes were gone. He had that unique odor that only burn victims radiate—the odor that every ED nurse can recognize. The clothes that remained were almost melted to his skin. Aside from the burns, the most obvious injury was a severe compound fracture of his right femur.

The emotional defenses we all possess as nurses immediately came into play as we approached the individual body part and specific task to which we were assigned. These defenses allow us to operate during the moment on specific tasks at hand. They allow for nurse and patient survival, in the moment. IV lines were started. Blood was sent. Portable x-rays were taken. Fluids were poured into every possible IV line. I went to work at his head.

I asked one of the people "What's his name?" To my surprise, I received the answer from our patient. He responded in a whispery, raspy voice—"Joey." I leaned down close to Joey's ear and told him "We're doing everything for you." He attempted a grin. The grin was quickly followed by a grimace as a colleague of mine punctured his skin to start another IV. I asked "Are you having much pain?" He bravely replied, "Some." My friend Gail and I had an instant between hasty activities to knowingly lock eyes. I yelled that we needed some morphine. A physician replied that we had to wait to check him neurologically. I said "Then now is the time to do it; he is awake and in pain."

I listened to Joey's lungs. The coarse sound indicated that he was burned internally as well. He coughed. Arterial blood gases were back. The oxygen mask would not be enough to keep his body oxygenated with the extent of his lung damage. His respirations became labored. An anesthesiologist arrived while I remained at Joey's head.

Joey opened his eyes and looked at me. I leaned closer and gently touched his face with my hand. In his hoarse voice he asked, "Will I be okay?" Gail glanced my way again. What to say? I hesitated for what seemed an eternity, then looked down at Joey and replied "We'll do everything we can to make sure you are okay, Joey." Despite the excruciating pain, his gaze caught mine and he attempted another grin. A tear formed in the corner of his eye and fell down the side of his face. He rasped "Thanks." Seconds later he was medicated to ease his pain. The anesthesiologist skillfully passed the tube through his vocal cords in order to ventilate his damaged lungs and oxygenate his body. Immediately he was whisked to the OR.

I learned that Joey died some time later. One never knows when the connection we make with someone will be his or her last.

Later, we learned that Joey had volunteered to help at a fair with the fireworks display. A Roman candle misfired and landed in the truck where Joey was unloading the other fireworks. Joey's family had been watching the display from their porch across a field and saw the truck explode.   ■

This story and the next are connected. Pat Reddish had a powerful and direct impact on my career. She was our psychiatric consultation liaison nurse in our large medical center where I worked in the cardiothoracic ICU. Her compassion, wisdom, and unique role inspired me. I later left critical care and pursued my masters in nursing, specializing in psychiatric consultation liaison nursing—to a large extent due to the influence of Pat.

When compiling stories for this book, I naturally sought my nursing mentors. Pat was one of these people. One of her prior secretaries helped me to find her. In our quest for contributors we sent sample vignettes. 'Joey' was a sample. I never knew, despite working at the same facility at the time, that Pat had even known about Joey until I received her contribution to this book, some 15 years after the incident.

These stories illustrate the unity of nursing as a healing force, and perhaps help to find meaning in tragedy.

—Jim Kane

Jim Kane, MN, RN, CS, CNAA
1978

JOEY'S FAMILY

In the early hours of the Fourth of July weekend I received a phone call from a nurse in the Burn Center. A teenage boy had been severely injured in a fireworks explosion. His parents and grandparents were in the waiting room. At that time they had no idea how devastating his injuries were. I was the psychiatric clinical nurse specialist for the critical care areas of a tertiary care hospital. My role was to provide crisis intervention for the patients and families. With only a psychiatric nursing background, I was truly a beginner. This was my first encounter with a major crisis. The intensity of the next 8 hours and the relationship that I developed with Joey's family would become the foundation of my learning about trauma, grief, and healing. More importantly, it taught me the meaning of being a nurse.

Joey died the next morning. I had asked his parents if they wanted to see him. They refused. They did not want to see the damaged body of their child. I was unsure so I did not force the issue.

Over the course of the next few months and years I maintained my relationship with the family. I referred them to self-help groups that dealt with the loss of a child. I helped them find a family therapist to assist the family in their grief. Joey's cousin Eddie had also been injured in the explosion. I referred Eddie to a child psychiatrist to help him cope with his own trauma and survivor's guilt. As time progressed they also shared happy events and milestones. I was invited to Eddie's homecoming after successful completion of Army basic training. I attended Grandpa's 80th birthday.

Our contacts lessened over the course of the next few years. Joey's parents became very active in the self-help group for parents who have lost children. I now referred families to them. They were always available to share their knowledge, sorrow, and hope with these families.

One afternoon in August 1986, Joey's parents called me and asked if they could see me within the next half-hour. They were at the county courthouse. Joey's lawsuit had just been resolved. When they arrived, we reviewed both the sadness and happiness experienced over the past 6 years. They were relieved and felt a sense of closure now that the legal proceedings were over. They wanted to return, for the last time, to the place where their child had died. My office was in the Burn Center. I had forgotten that his parents had never been in the unit. As they were leaving his mother said "Joey was in Room 15, wasn't he?" I was surprised and asked her how she knew. She said, "I was too afraid to see him but I was with him. I hope you've always made a mother be with her child before he dies, no matter what."

This final visit was a powerful reminder of how we as nurses are permitted entry into those most intimate moments of people's lives. Joey's family permitted me to share their lives. They taught me about the intensity and endurance of grief. They also taught me that healing and hope endure. They helped me to develop objectivity, empathy, and skills to help other families facing these devastating moments. They showed me that a nurse could heal wounds that can't be seen. ∎

Patricia Reddish, MSN, RN, CS
1980

SALLY AND PETE

During my first month as a community health nurse in the Bronx, I found myself at the door in a dingy hallway. From behind the door I heard a dog bark, a loud bell, and muffled voices. Nervously, I awaited the opening of the door. Suddenly the door flew open and a short woman, about 75 years old, stood in front of me holding the barking dog. Speaking with a nasal tone to her voice she uttered "Um in." I stepped inside and saw wires running along the walls attached to bell boxes and flashing lights. The wires followed a course through all the rooms which, though spotlessly clean, had limited furnishings.

The woman, Sally, kept uttering nasal sounds. She tried telling me a story about her husband, but I couldn't understand her. I kept saying "I'm the nurse, where is Peter?" She grabbed my arm and directed me toward the bedroom. Peter sat on the side of a twin bed, hunched over with his arms outstretched on a bedside table.

"Hi, I'm your patient" the man said clearly. "I'm blind and my wife is deaf. We use the dog as an alerting system. The wires you see connect to flashing lights and a bell system, which goes off when the door bell or phone rings. I rigged

the system myself," he added proudly.

Peter was 75 years old, with severe chronic pulmonary lung disease. As I checked his vital signs, he told me his life story. Blinded at an early age, he was determined to be independent. He used to walk every day to the subways and take the train to Manhattan. He met Sally, married, and they had two children, neither of whom came by to visit or help. That was okay, he said, because he knew how to survive and take care of himself and Sally.

He then told me about his most recent hospital stay, which he described as 'horrible.' He had been placed on a ventilator and said people thought he must be stupid because he was blind. And, when they saw Sally, they really would not listen to either of them, believing them to be nonfunctional.

I was to evaluate his respiratory status, teach him to use the nebulizer, and instruct both of them about his medications. He listened as I methodically went down the list.

After the first few medications I said, "How are you going to know when and how to take your medicines, even if I pour them out in the Mediset?" Sally watched every move I made since I entered her domain. Peter said, "Sally will take care of it." She could read lips somewhat, but she mainly watched what I did and repeated with her nasal voice the task of how to distribute the medications. I felt a little uneasy leaving them. "How could they possibly manage?" I thought.

The next day as my supervisor and I stood in front of the door, I explained the signal of the barking dog. The door flew open and Sally, who looked in a frenzy, said "Quick! Quick!" We ran into the bedroom and Peter was in the midst of an asthma attack. As I checked Peter's vital signs, my supervisor told the patient we would have to call 911. In between gasps he said, "I don't want to go on any machines." Sally concurred, "No machines, no machines." I wanted to respect his wishes, and yet I knew if he went to the ER in an ambulance and the situation remained severe, the physicians would most likely put Peter on a ventilator.

As the ambulance personnel entered the home, some of them snickered at all the 'contraptions.' They secured Peter onto the stretcher and I heard him whimpering between breaths, "No machines, no machines."

The ambulance crew would not let Sally into the ambulance and she began donning her coat.

"How are you going to get to the hospital?" I asked.

She looked at me with tears in her eyes, "Walk." I could feel her fear. If she got there too late, who would listen to a blind man saying he doesn't want life support?

"I'll drive you" I said. "I can't help it. I must do this." Off we went to the ER and arrived some time after Peter. The physicians and nurses were hovering over Peter's stretcher. Sally burst in, yelling in her nasal twang, "No machines, no machines." But they had just intubated Peter and were about to attach him to the machine.

As they wheeled Peter to his room, Sally and I watched in tears. As Peter went by she grabbed him and hugged him. Tears flowed from his eyes, too.

After dropping Sally off back at her home, I felt so helpless. Here was a couple who had both worked, managed to live on their own, and function without help from anyone—and their voices went unheard.

Each day, as I walked my 'beat' in the neighborhood, I'd run into Sally. She'd hold on to my arm and walk with me to the apartment buildings and update me on the latest happenings in the hospital with Peter. People around us stared, for many of the neighborhood regulars thought her to be insane. I knew differently, for I had been granted access to their hidden world.

A week later, I was standing in front of Pete and Sally's door. Pete had made it through another episode with the machine. The familiar dog signaled my arrival. When the door flew open Sally grabbed me and hugged me saying "Es ome, es ome." I knew this, of course, since I had been referred to see him again.

Karen Bauer, MS, RN
1982

56

MARIE

It was after the Thanksgiving holiday when I was asked to see Marie. I was a psychiatric liaison clinical nurse specialist who saw physically ill patients experiencing some type of emotional discomfort—from normal grief reaction to severe psychosis. I was called by the medical intensive care nursing staff to 'talk to' Marie, who recently had been admitted with a diagnosis of Guillian-Barré syndrome: an autoimmune disorder that appears like flu, with fever, muscle aches, and fatigue, and progresses to paralysis of the muscles.

Marie's Guillian-Barré syndrome had progressed swiftly from her flu-like symptoms, which lasted 3 weeks, until her paralysis. Her paralysis was almost complete; she could not breathe on her own and a respirator was breathing for her. The staff nurses and physicians caring for Marie believed her to be depressed because of her illness and she had been prescribed antidepressants.

Marie was a 50-year-old nurse who had worked in rehabilitation nursing at one time. She was married and had two children—a daughter and a son who were both married. This sudden illness had taken her by surprise. As I entered the room to see Marie, I noticed that she was quite alert, almost fearful as she gazed at this new person approaching her. When I introduced myself and told her why I was there, it became apparent to me why she was so frightened. She could not talk and she could not use her hands or head to gesture— therefore, communicating was extremely difficult. Although she could not talk, Marie could 'mouth the words,' though no sound would come out because of the respirator tube down her throat.

As I talked to Marie and began my assessment of Marie's depression, I noticed that her eyes kept darting to the bulletin board, which had listed all the latest x-ray results, blood values, oxygen levels, and prescribed medications. Her eyes also darted to the ceiling and to the window. After I did my usual orientation check to see if Marie knew where she was, who she was, and why she was in the hospital, I asked her, "Marie, are you having any 'bad dreams' or seeing anything that is disturbing you?" Marie looked at me and mouthed "yes." I sat closer to her and asked "Tell me what you see." Marie immediately looked frightened and said "There are people out the window laughing and pointing at me. They are angry with me. There are men above me and animals who mean to do me harm."

As a psychiatric liaison nurse, I was thinking to myself that she is clearly hallucinating and no wonder she is so frightened. Since the medical intensive care unit was on the fifth floor, I told Marie that there were no people out the window or on the ceiling, but that a medication that she was taking could be causing her to hallucinate. I talked with the physicians and nursing staff about stopping the antidepressants since they would be ineffective at this time in Marie's illness.

I came back to check on Marie the next day and was rewarded by a less frightened lady. She remained anxious about her disease and whether she would regain the use of her body, but she was not hallucinating. This was the beginning of our year-long relationship. It took Marie 4 months before she could breathe without the respirator and was moved out of the intensive care unit. She spent another 3 months preparing to go to rehabilitation, where she would relearn how to walk and use her hands. We continued to meet and discuss her psychological recovery, as well.

During these talks, Marie taught me a lot about being a patient and I asked her if she would mind videotaping her story so that I could use it to educate medical students and psychiatric residents. Marie, in her unassuming way, said "What do I have to offer any student that they do not already know?" I replied, "More than you will ever know."

It was during the videotaping of her story that Marie looked at me seriously and said "You were the first person who took the time to look at me in the face and take the time to communicate with me when I was so frightened. You were the one who asked the most uncomfortable questions about seeing 'things.' I was so afraid that the staff would put me away in a psychiatric hospital. But you were there to comfort me, to talk to me, and to make me aware of what was happening to me. The most important thing that I can tell students is to communicate directly with the patient. Don't ask how the person is doing while you read the machines. Look at the person when you are talking."

I now teach undergraduate and graduate nursing students and show them the video of Marie. I often think of Marie and how much she taught me. Now I use Marie's story to teach other nurses and health professionals how important it is to communicate face-to-face with the patient and take time to listen to the person. ■

Jane Bryant Neese, PhD, RN, CS
1987

PEI JUN

"I am wrong, I am wrong." Those words, uttered in Chinese, are what Pei Jun, a 22-year-old rural woman, would repeat many times each day while crying and kowtowing on the ward where I was psych co-head nurse. I had been living at a psychiatric hospital in central China for the past 5 years. Initially, I had come to the hospital to teach English so I could be with my fiance, a Canadian psychiatrist/anthropologist. Over time, he and I became the co-directors of the teaching ward on which Pei Jun was hospitalized.

This was her fifth psychiatric hospitalization since the age of 16. Diagnosed with schizophrenia, Pei Jun had symptoms of anxiety, poor appetite, delusions of sin and guilt, running away from home, and hearing voices of her uncle cursing and degrading her. At the age of 13, she was raped by her uncle. She had told her parents but they would not believe her and denied that the rape had happened. Just prior to this hospitalization she had been rejected by a boyfriend when he learned that she was not a virgin.

Because of her frequent illness relapses and unresponsiveness to medication, her Chinese doctor asked me to talk with her. As she was crying on her bed I approached her, sat down beside her, and touched her. Usually Chinese nurses do not sit on a patient's bed or touch patients purely for comfort. I began by telling her how hard it must be for her to have had something so awful happen to her. And I let her cry. Then I said, if anyone were to be blamed for what happened, it would be her uncle. "You were a young girl. You could not resist your uncle. What happened was not your fault." Pei Jun stopped crying momentarily and looked at me. Her face was a mixture of disbelief and hope.

I met with Pei Jun daily for the next 5 days, repeating the same message. During these days she underwent a remarkable change. This was the first time someone had acknowledged that she was not responsible for the rape. Her schizophrenic symptoms disappeared. She stopped crying, interacted with other patients, and began talking of her future plans for finding a spouse. Her doctor and other staff members were amazed at the transformation. Within 2 weeks she was discharged from the hospital.

Eight months later I saw her again. She was happy and had returned to work. The burdens of guilt and shame were lifted from her shoulders. She had been set free. ∎

Marlys Bueber, MN, RN, CNS
1993

MICHAEL

Michael was his parents' pride and joy, an unexpected 'gift of life' given to them in their later years. At age 18 he was considered a model person on the brink of adulthood. He had a wonderful summer job, his own set of wheels, and a full scholarship to USC, which he would attend in the fall. His parents were bursting with pride over their only child's remarkable accomplishments and the young man he had become.

In the summer of his 18th year, Michael was returning home from work. It was late. A drunken driver at the wheel of a large sedan recklessly ran through a red light, veered off course, and struck Michael's Volkswagen Bug head-on. The impact thrust Michael's head against the windshield. Paramedics at the scene found him unconscious and unresponsive. They quickly initiated resuscitation measures and rushed him to the nearest trauma center. Despite aggressive treatment and all the modern medical technology available to these skilled trauma surgeons, Michael remained totally unresponsive.

Afterwards, Michael was transferred to the trauma ICU where I was assigned. He was intubated and comatose and receiving intravenous fluids and vasopressor drugs to maintain his blood pressure and organ perfusion.

His CAT scan revealed a massive brain stem injury with other areas of the brain also compromised. Unfortunately, despite the efforts of the neurosurgical team, relieving the abnormally high intracranial pressure was simply not enough to stimulate spontaneous respiration. Since Michael's coma continued and EEGs showed no activity in his brain, Michael was pronounced clinically dead. As a result, all other body functions were maintained through life support systems, anticipating parental approval for organ procurement.

At that time, I was a novice critical care nurse. Because I was not married and had no children, my colleagues deemed me to be the most appropriate nurse to care for Michael. I was overwhelmed at the prospect of explaining and supporting Michael's grief-stricken parents through this process.

Michael's parents had followed his gurney into the ICU. At first I thought they were Michael's grandparents. His father's hair was sparse and completely gray, the lines on his face were deepened into crevices, and grief creased his forehead. Michael's mother was diminutive and frail.

Michael's parents stood patiently by his side as I busied myself performing the physiological aspects of care needed to maintain Michael's organs. Diligently, I was repeatedly in and out of his room, regulating his IV fluid, continually adjusting the dopamine infusion and ventilator settings, while closely monitoring his vital signs and urine output. In my frenzy I lost track of how long Michael's parents hovered over him. When I finally stopped, I looked up and found myself gazing directly into the eyes of Michael's father. Many questions were apparent there, but I was frightened to initiate that discussion. I searched my soul for the appropriate words and suddenly, without conscious thought, heard myself whisper, "Would you like to pray?"

Michael's father remained silent for a long moment. Finally he looked upward beyond the ceiling and prayed with a spirit of humility. He thanked God for his gift of 18 wonderful years with this incredible child. Then he took his wife's hand, touched my arm expressively, and departed.

His gift of love, understanding, and refusal to condemn God in these truly unexplainable circumstances will remain an inspiration upon my heart forever. ∎

Lori L. Burnell, MSN, RN
1978

THE SMITH FAMILY

I work in a pediatric clinic providing health care services to a variety of clients. One day I noted that the next patients on my schedule were two little boys ages 4 and 5. They were at the clinic for a physical because they were brothers and had just been placed in a new foster home. The state requires a physical exam on all children within a week of being placed in a foster home. I walked into the room and encountered two little boys who were literally climbing the walls. They could not sit still for even a few seconds. It didn't take me long to feel exasperated with these two children. I looked in utter amazement at the foster parents, wondering how long anyone could tolerate these two boys in their house.

The foster parents were two men, Ted and Ray. They were a gay couple who had been referred to me by a friend of theirs who brought his granddaughter to me for her care. I spent a great deal of time taking as detailed a history from these two men as they could give me. They were in a stable long-term relationship. They wanted children and knew that the only way they could become parents was to become foster parents. They were both employed in good jobs and were willing to make any sacrifices necessary to become parents.

The boys' social situation was dismal. They were the 5th and 6th children born to a drug-addicted mother who had given up custody of all of her children. The boys had been in and out of foster homes since birth. They suffered from severe attention deficit disorder and were considered unadoptable because their behavior was so bad. This had been music to the ears of Ted and Ray, who wanted to adopt this set of brothers and create a family.

I was skeptical. I spent a great deal of time talking to Ted and Ray about how many obstacles they would be facing (as if they didn't know!). Having an instant family could spell disaster to even a 'normal,' stable relationship with 'normal' children. These men faced what appeared to be insurmountable odds. The two little boys were going to be very difficult to live with. I doubted they could do it, but I told them I would be there for them no matter what.

The next 2 years brought them to my office many times. I listened while they talked about the many adjustments they had to make as they bought a house. I listened while they discussed having to change their work schedules—one working evenings and one working during the day—so that one of them was available to go to school with the boys. I listened while they discussed how much stress they were under and what a strain it was on their relationship. I listened while they discussed that the court was examining every detail of their lives while they tried to adopt these two children. Ted and Ray wanted to provide more for these boys than just food and a roof over their heads. They wanted to be able to tell them they would never have to have another set of parents again.

I watched in amazement while these two boys were transformed from difficult, unruly children, to well-behaved, loving boys. I took care of them when they came in with asthma, and recommended a counselor while we adjusted medication to help the boys in school. I found myself considering asking Ted and Ray if they would give parenting classes for some of my other patients because they were the best parents I had in my practice. One of the men always came with the boys for every appointment. They called me to discuss the small successes and the large frustrations.

Recently I looked on my schedule and found I had a walk-in appointment with the boys. When I walked into the exam room, I was informed by both boys that they had a very special surprise for me. I couldn't wait to hear what they wanted to share with me. They had brought me the pictures from the courthouse, immediately after their adoption. Ray and Ted had changed the last names of the boys at the time of the adoption. The boys proudly informed me that they were now the 'Smith family.' I gave everyone a hug and told both boys I thought they had the best family in the whole world! Both men looked at me. They did not need to say thank you. I could see it in the eyes of everyone present.

I was touched beyond words that they wanted me to share this important moment with them. It is not very often that you can be present at the birth of a new and special family. ■

Renee P. McLeod, MSN, RN, CPNP
1998

MRS. SANSON

"I can't carry on a conversation with her. She's bizarre. Being around her gives me the creeps."

The staff pleaded, "Do something with her, please." Since this group of nurses was not hesitant to tackle difficult situations, I paid attention. They were consistently responsive to problem-solving a perplexing patient or family scenario. We then collectively shared our expertise— their critical care nursing skills and my mental health skills—with the patient or family. The nurses quickly described Mrs. Sanson. She came to the ICU wearing dark sunglasses, eccentrically attired, and offering few words. She spoke only when asked a direct question. "She doesn't make sense when she talks."

I walked to the family waiting room and found it empty except for the woman I identified from their descriptions. I introduced myself as a nurse who worked with the ICU staff and indicated I was aware her husband was quite ill.

Because the dark glasses obscured Mrs. Sanson's eyes, I found it difficult to determine if she looked at me when I asked how she was doing. It was my hunch, however, that she also had a chronic psychiatric condition; but since she was not our patient, the goal was not to treat it. Our role was to assist her through the course of her husband's illness and impending death.

I kept this initial visit brief. I let Mrs. Sanson know we wanted to support her at the same time we attended to her husband. I sensed both her surprise and relief. Then I garnered her permission to talk again the following day.

Entering the waiting room late the next morning, I saw her again sitting alone. This time I saw her raise her head as I said "Hello, Mrs. Sanson."

"Hello," she echoed, without giving me eye contact.

"May I sit down?" I asked. She nodded affirmatively. As I took my place in a chair near her, I noticed she was picking at the brightly colored material of the skirt she wore. Her blouse was also garish and a complete mismatch with the skirt. Dark glasses covered her eyes. Sitting on top of her head was a hat that complemented neither blouse nor skirt. I started by asking what she understood about her husband's condition. "He's very sick" she said. As we continued, her responses to my queries were sometimes completely inappropriate to the question. When this occurred I simply said "What you just said doesn't make sense to me, Mrs. Sanson." I simply made the comment and proceeded with the conversation.

I commented on how difficult it must be for her to have a husband so ill. I said "It must make you wonder whether he will survive this illness." She sighed and nodded her head slightly.

"He's probably done a lot to manage things in your lives, hasn't he?"

"Everything," she said without looking up. I paused for a moment before venturing, "It's hard for me to talk while you're wearing those dark glasses. It would really help me if you could take them off." After a long pause, Mrs. Sanson slowly raised one hand to the glasses, removed them, and placed them in her lap.

"Thank you, Mrs. Sanson. I appreciate your doing that." Her action supported my hunch that she knew I sincerely wanted to help.

Over the next few days I continued to meet with Mrs. Sanson. Each day she arrived with her sunglasses in place, but removed them once in the unit. This simple change affected the ICU staff, who now engaged with her each time she came to her husband's bedside. I noticed each nurse stood next to her and touched her husband while the conversation occurred. I also began to see Mrs. Sanson place her hand over her husband's. Although there was no reaction from Mr. Sanson, I could see a softening in Mrs. Sanson's eyes when she looked at him.

I ventured into an area that I knew needed addressing: I indicated her husband might not survive. Mrs. Sanson stopped fidgeting. She softly said "I know." In a rambling, somewhat incoherent style, she started to describe how much she

relied on him. His unexpected illness unsettled her terribly. She knew he wasn't getting better. She couldn't talk to him. She took the bus to the hospital each day but felt she could do nothing to help him.

Slowly, gently, but quite directly, I addressed our concern for her should something happen to her husband. I asked if she had anyone. She said "No." Then her expression lightened and she said "I have a social worker." It seems she also took medicine for "her condition."

"I wonder if I call could this social worker, Mrs. Sanson? I could explain what's happening here."

"You would do that?" she asked without looking. I said "Yes, I would."

I was grateful for the few days to build this relationship with Mrs. Sanson. Somehow I had the feeling her husband was hanging on until we could do something to help his wife.

Her social worker was unaware of Mr. Sanson's hospitalization for this life-threatening illness. She thanked me for telephoning and assured me she would call Mrs. Sanson. Mr. Sanson had managed all their affairs.

The next morning Mr. Sanson died. I found Mrs. Sanson in a shadowed corner of the waiting room. She did not look up. I saw no tears. After expressing my condolences, I accompanied her downstairs to the person who helps with arrangements.

While I introduced the clerk to Mrs. Sanson, she was appropriate in both conversation and expression throughout the exchange. I offered to call the social worker to see if she could come to get her. Mrs. Sanson declined, saying that she would be able to take the bus home. I said I'd call the social worker to let her know of her husband's death. "I'll be OK" she said, as if to reassure me. In the lobby, she stood next to me for a moment, turned, extended her hand to shake mine, and said "Thank you." I remember it to this day because she looked directly into my eyes. ∎

Donna Ehrenreich, MN, RN, CS
1981

JOHN AND GREG

In 1978, as an experienced critical care-turned cardiac rehab nurse, I worked with a couple who remain vivid in my memory. They taught me about love, courage, and generosity of spirit.

John had a heart attack at the age of 52. After reviewing his chart, I went to the bedside for our first visit. We began to talk about his symptoms, how he was feeling at the moment and what he thought the impact would be upon his life. While we were talking, visiting hours began. A very attractive man came into the room. He introduced himself as Greg and sat down at the bedside. John and I chatted for a few minutes more and agreed to meet the next afternoon to discuss discharge plans and risk factor modification. I suggested that it would be helpful if a family member could be there to hear the information as well.

When I entered the room the next afternoon at our scheduled time, Greg again was sitting at the bedside. We talked for a few minutes and I asked John if any family members would be joining us. He glanced at the younger man sitting beside him, looked up at me and said "Greg is my family."

"Okay," I replied, being perky in that annoying, young, know-it-all

fashion. "He can't possibly be your son, you're much too young. Is he your brother?"

John looked seriously at me, probably astounded at my naïveté, and said, "Greg is my lover. We've been together for 10 years."

I was taken aback. I grew up in the southern United States where homosexuality was still not widely accepted, and I had not been introduced to an openly gay person until college. I had, as far as I knew, no gay friends and would not have been much more surprised had John claimed to be a Martian! I did manage to pull my foot out of my mouth and begin the first of our discussions about cardiac anatomy, physiology, and risk factors.

In the late 70s, MI patients were routinely kept in the hospital for 10 days. As the days passed, John, Greg, and I spoke frequently. We discussed risk factor modification, exercise, diet, medications, cardiac signs and symptoms. I encouraged them to participate in the hospital's cardiac rehabilitation program. We got to know one another and I saw the deep care and concern that they had for one another, the gentleness that they expressed in little ways as a couple. I was moved and enlarged as a person by observing how they interacted. They were like any loving, committed couple with whom I worked.

As the discharge day approached, I found myself avoiding one topic that routinely was discussed with cardiac patients. Usually, I had no difficulty talking to patients about sexual activity. I had discussed sex with men older than my father and 20-something, single and married people, but never with anyone who was gay.

One afternoon, when I came into the room, John looked at me, smiled, and reached for Greg's hand. He took a deep breath and said, "I know this is probably uncomfortable for you, but we need to talk about sex. What can't we do, what can we do, and when?"

I was simultaneously touched by their courage in pursuing the information they needed, and embarrassed by my discomfort. Their concern for my feelings should have been unnecessary. They put me at ease with their openness and empathy. We discussed their usual sexual practices and although I had no readily available resource materials to help, we spoke of general principles. I promised to investigate further and get additional information. We were able to find appropriate advice to share with them and clarify their questions. Whenever I got tongue-tied at not knowing exactly how to discuss something, John or Greg would help me.

John was discharged in good condition with a good prognosis. He attended our cardiac rehabilitation program for a few months, and I was able to see his physical condition improve steadily. Psychologically, John moved through the same adjustments as anyone with a major illness. But he spoke often to me of how Greg's support was helping him through the emotional ups and downs of recovery. John returned to work and, the last I knew, was living well with his disease under control in the same loving, committed relationship.

I don't believe that I was prejudiced in 1978, but gay people were outside my conscious experience, different. . .unknown. John and Greg gave me a tremendous gift, to see individuals who were different from me and ask "Are these good people? Do they care for one another and for others?"

I have met many, many people since who are different in one way or another, as we all are. We are all part of the tapestry of humankind, rich with color and texture. Although my mother, who is also a nurse, tried to explain it with words as we grew up, it was demonstrated fully by two wonderful men who hugged me one afternoon and said "It wasn't so hard, was it? Thanks!" I hugged them back and replied, "Thank YOU." ∎

Donna Nolten, MN, RN, C, CNA
1978

COLLEAGUES

The day seemed slow and uneventful to me this quiet Sunday afternoon. Theresa was completely the opposite, since she was preoccupied with the anticipation of her first child. He was already 10 days late. Rubbing her swollen abdomen she felt a twinge of anxiety when the phone rang. The nurse midwife said "I was looking at your ultrasound again and that boy seems large and ready to be born. It's slow today, would you like to come in and be induced?" Theresa, a nurse herself, knew about the procedure she was to encounter.

The drive to the hospital was exciting. Theresa talked about her delight and joy with her husband. She felt supported and safe, thinking "What could be better than having a psychologist as a Lamaze coach?"

Theresa entered the hospital and was asked to sit in a wheelchair. She felt odd. She was accustomed to being in control in medical situations. She felt this strangeness repeatedly as they started the IV and injected Pitocin.

The contractions began. Her loving husband tried to soothe her. Every relaxation technique was attempted without success. She began ordering her husband around

and finally sent him out of the room. The nurses watched patiently. Some were intimidated and left as soon as their task was done.

One, however, had the courage to enter her world of pain and loss of control. She approached Theresa and said "I know what you're going through; it's not easy being a patient when you're a nurse." The nurse sat by Theresa and said nothing. She waited. Theresa finally said "help me." It was then that the relationship began and the journey into motherhood became a little easier. The nurse gave her permission to cry out, to give up all control, and to be vulnerable.

The time seemed endless for Theresa as she labored. The pain was excruciating, yet bearable, as the nurse broke through the barriers and successfully helped Theresa to relax. Theresa remembers the stroking of her head, wiping the perspiration from her brow, singing, the smell of her perfume, and her quiet, patient, accepting voice. They tried everything together: breathing, squatting, grunting, laughing for brief moments, and story-telling. What Theresa remembers most was her devotion, patience, and loyalty. What she still wishes she could remember about this nurse is her *name*.

Theresa believes that she would not have been able to persevere with the labor and delivery had it not been for her. She is inspired, having witnessed a colleague in action and benefitted from her expertise and caring. Theresa will be forever grateful and pass on the collegial tenderness whenever possible. ∎

Jan Cipkala-Gaffin, MN, RN, CS
1986

BARB

Healthcare is a world of its own. Healthcare professionals have their own language and systems. Generally, the public seems curious about us. They want to know a little but not too much. Most of all, they want to know that we are there for them when they need us. It is a challenge for us healthcare workers to take a frightened, anxious, sick person and turn that person back into a healthy, functioning human being. Yet when that challenge is accomplished, it's a great feeling for all involved. The process occurs through education, skill, and empowerment. Barb was yet another patient who reinforced this notion.

Barb had a poorly functioning bladder that required surgery. The surgeons added a piece of intestine to the top of her bladder so it would store urine appropriately. She would now have to learn how to catheterize herself to drain urine from her bladder. Barb asked a lot of questions, which is always a good sign. It was difficult to try to describe the difference between bowel versus intestine versus colon. However, it was important for her to know the anatomy of her new urinary system. She was obviously anxious about learning to self-catheterize. With a lot of coaching and cheerleading, she was able to

do it. You could see the pride and relief on her face.

It takes a while for patients to establish trust in their caregivers. Once that trust is established, patients are able to discuss their true feelings, and that is often when we can make a difference. Barb vented her feelings of frustration to me. She felt that the doctors didn't take the time to explain things to her. I listened and applauded her on her assertiveness to learn everything about her medical condition. I explained, however, that it is not only the doctors who can provide her with the information that she needed. We discussed the other healthcare team members and their roles in helping her get both the care and the education she required.

I guess when I told her she had the right to be informed and to manage her situation, she decided to give me her two cents on my performance. Barb explained to me that she was dissatisfied that I had nursing students working with her without asking her first. Once again, Barb pointed out to me something that I probably just take for granted. I explained to her that most of us assume it is okay for students to work with patients because she was being cared for in a teaching hospital. I thanked her for her openness and promised to try to keep this in mind with her and other patients in the future.

Later that day I was talking with Barb's surgical intern, Elaine. We discussed Barb's progress and the further care she would need. During the discussion we were snacking on a fudgy chocolate cake in the conference room. Elaine started chuckling. The humor was contagious and I started laughing with her as I asked, "What's so funny?" Elaine told me about how the senior residents had played a few practical jokes on her during her residency. "How can I get some of this cake on the bottom of their shoes or on the back of their lab coats?" she asked as she laughed. I had to admit, this cake did look like you-know-what. We both were getting giddy and started brainstorming on how to retaliate.

A thought suddenly came to me and I jumped up and ran to the storage room. I took an emesis basin and smooshed some of the cake and toilet paper into it. I instructed Elaine to follow me. We went down to Barb's room. We both knew her well and decided to have her participate in the joke. Laughter can be the best medicine. I said to Barb, "Hey Barb, how would you like to play a little practical joke with us on the residents?" Barb was excited and said "Sure." I filled her in on the plan. We three were so goofy with laughter we could hardly wait to see it carried out.

Later that evening the surgical team (the attending, the residents, and Elaine) rounded on Barb. They started with the traditional "How is everything going?" Barb reported to

them her success at self-catheterization. They talked about her plans to go home. Barb then explained that she had a question. She reached over for the basin that we had placed on her side table. "How come my stool looks different than before my surgery?" she asked. The residents and attending physicians looked a little perplexed as to why a patient would have stool in this manner. They immediately, however, went into the explanation about how they used the bowel to make the bladder bigger and maybe the bowel hadn't adjusted yet. Barb said "Oh." Barb then dipped her finger into the 'stool,' put it in her mouth, and said, "Then why does it taste different than my stool before surgery?" By this time Elaine was bursting at the seams and could no longer hold in the laughter when she saw the look of shock on the residents' faces! Barb and Elaine explained it was a joke and everyone laughed.

When you work with a well-established team, including the patient, you can accomplish great things and have fun doing it. Although our having Barb participate might be considered risky, it actually served to empower her by providing a chance to communicate in a different way with the team and practice her newfound assertiveness as a health care consumer. ∎

Susan Allison, MS, RN, CS, CETN
1996

JUDY

I had worked with Judy for several months while doing a stint as a per diem hospice nurse. Judy was a librarian. She smoked and was now dying of lung cancer. Typical of hospice relationships, Judy and I wasted little time getting down to discussing the reality of her terminal illness. In particular, Judy wanted to know about suicide. We discussed all aspects of suicide.

Frequently during my visits, the conversation would turn to her suicide. Judy asked if I would assist her when the right time came. I always have believed in assisted suicide theoretically, particularly for the terminally ill. I have never been asked to assist, or expected to do it. However, I would nod positively, while silently praying I would never have to follow through. As luck would have it, I got a different job and left per diem hospice nursing. It was particularly tough for me to say good-bye to Judy. There was something very genuine about her. Perhaps it was Judy's courage or bravery.

Every day or so, after I changed jobs, I would think of Judy and wonder how she was doing. Occasionally we would talk on the phone and always the subject of suicide would come up. As always, I agreed I would assist her. Many sleepless hours were spent

wondering how I would get around this complex mess. It was very much against the agency policy to even discuss suicide with a patient. I had long ago broken that rule. In addition, any patients discussing suicide were to be immediately referred for psychiatric evaluation. I had never acknowledged on any document our discussions about suicide. I felt a certain patient confidentiality with Judy regardless of the consequences. I understood her perspective.

One morning, several months later, the phone rang; it was Judy. Judy chatted away for a few moments and then asked if I could come visit her. She sounded fine and said she missed talking to me. I thought to myself, "Oh God, now what do I do?" Nonetheless, I immediately said "Yes." We made arrangements for me to visit that afternoon. The rest of the day I was a wreck. I kept thinking, "What if she asks me, what am I going to do?"

I got to the apartment where she was living. Estelle, her friend, let me in. Judy was sitting up in 'her' chair smoking a cigarette. We talked. Judy seemed tired of the ordeal, wondering aloud to me "How long was this going to go on? I'm so tired." I kept anticipating her big question, "Would I help her?" The question never came up.

Judy was having some serious complications due to her illness. I decided to encourage Judy to spend 1 or 2 days as a hospice inpatient so that some palliative measures could be initiated. Judy was terribly reluctant, but had finally agreed to be admitted.

While I was on the phone making the necessary arrangements, Judy got up, walked to the bathroom, came back, sat down and had another cigarette. As things typically go, the admission for palliative treatment was taking some time. Judy looked at me and said "I really feel terrible." At first I just looked at her, but realized quickly that something was happening. I told the woman with whom I was speaking to hold on, and I went to Judy. I was holding her and rubbing her back. Judy looked at me and then started to bleed profusely from her mouth. I gently eased her to the floor as she continued to bleed. I felt very calm. I knew that Judy was going to die. Judy just quietly, so quietly, so peacefully continued to bleed, then died.

I don't remember talking much. I do, however, remember a great urge and need to call 911 and try to 'save' her. It was an odd feeling of great conflict. Should I try to save her? Why? Judy was terminally ill. Or did I just want to save me? All the talk about death and dying was happening right now. Everything I believed in, or thought I believed in was being challenged. I finally realized that Judy had known and trusted me to let her go, to be there with her and for her, and not to try to save her the traditional way, but to just let it happen.

I was so struck by her sharing this incredible experience with me. How was it possible that I was there with her when she died? I felt Judy had honored me by sharing her death with me. I felt privileged to be a part of Judy's death. I was able to assist Judy in her dying, but surely not the way I had feared. I helped in a far more meaningful and spiritual way—maybe she knew all along. Since this incredible experience, I have been honored and unafraid to be with many people at the time of their death. Thank you Judy. ■

Maggie Finch, MA, RN
1989

GAYE

Fall semester, I had a group of students on a cardiology unit. Gaye was one of those students. She was slightly older than the others, was from England, and had been an LPN, who was seeking to become an RN. When I watched her with patients, I knew she was someone very special. She had a quiet peace and listened attentively to her patients, reassuring them with her calm and quiet humor.

Gaye came to my office one day and was obviously upset. I was alarmed because Gaye usually took most situations in stride. Her eyes welled up with tears while she spoke with me. "Judy, I don't know what to do." I encouraged her to continue, "My mum is sick back home. She has cancer and is dying. I want to be with her but my mum's greatest wish is for me to finish my education and she wouldn't want me to come home to care for her if it would cause me not to finish my studies."

"Gaye, I can see this is tearing you apart. You would always regret not being with your mother during her final days. I think we can arrange it so you can finish clinical and be with your mother."

It was agreed that Gaye would finish her clinical rotation when she returned from England. Gaye spent the next couple of months at home

Judy Cohen, PhD, RN
1987

and returned after her mother had died. Although saddened, Gaye was at peace with herself. I supervised the rest of her clinical rotation on cardiology during semester break and she finished up her studies with the rest of the class.

Often we don't realize the profound effect we are having on one another in a caring relationship. For as much as I might have had an impact on Gaye, she had an equally powerful effect on me almost 12 years later. My own beloved father was on a cardiology unit being evaluated for chest pain after an illness. Gaye was the nurse on the unit. She saw me visit him daily and witnessed his 89th birthday. She was always there showing concern and offering a reassuring word.

My father died 3 weeks later and Gaye sent me a note. "I read your dad's obituary. I hope that yesterday's services proved to be both a wonderful tribute as well as a celebration of his life. I could see and feel your pain as you came to grips with the reality of the situation. I could also see what a pillar of strength you obviously are to your mum. So hope that the happy memories of your dad soon overshadow the ones surrounding his illness and death. A wonderful coping mechanism that I discovered after losing my mum is to acknowledge some little thing every single day that I know would have given her pleasure. Somehow it always helps me to feel close to her and keep her lovely memory alive. Will look forward very much to seeing you again on the unit with students soon." ∎

EDDIE

I was working in two roles on an acute psychiatric unit. Half the time I was an inservice educator and half the time a staff nurse. It was a teaching hospital and once a year all the doctors change. This occurred right after the annual change.

Eddie was an interesting man. He had served successfully for 2 years in the military, had earned one of the highest math scores on a college entrance exam, and had a very chronic and difficult disease. Eddie had schizophrenia and was out of touch with reality most of the time. Eddie had a childlike quality, kind of like a 14-year-old who never made it out of puberty. He was messy in appearance, in love with me (and several other nurses as well), and didn't like taking medication for his disease. Taking it every day means "I'm sick and I don't want to be or feel sick" and the side effects are 'lousy.'

Eddie had been in the hospital 2 or 3 times that spring. It was now summer and one more medication was being used. The medication change seemed to be a success—Eddie was pretty clear. I recommended to the new doctors that he move to the less restrictive open unit and he did.

One day when I was functioning as the educator, Eddie wanted a craft and slippers (he rarely wore shoes). I got both for him, told him I'd see him later, and left the unit. Eddie killed himself that day. He left the unit, signed out for a walk, and crossed the street to a tall building and jumped.

Eddie left a note about no more meds to try. Despite my intellectual rationalizing about the high mortality rate of mental illness, I cried a lot, felt responsible and helpless, and almost quit psychiatric nursing.

I went to Eddie's memorial service where his mother greeted me and told me what a difference I had made in Eddie's life. She went on to say she believed he was happier now and how much it meant to her for me to attend the funeral.

Thank you Eddie, for the lessons. Thank you Eddie's Mom—I would have missed a great deal, not to mention interesting people, if I had left nursing. ∎

Ann Kelly, MSN, RN, CS
1991

MARIA'S
NEIGHBORS

In the winter, the Bronx, New York, can be a cold, forbidding place. Especially when you have just had your first baby and your family is living in Puerto Rico. That was how Maria was feeling the day I visited her for the first time after receiving a referral from the maternity clinic at a local hospital. Maria had recently joined her husband Jose, who was a short-order cook at the local diner. Jose worked long hours and Maria felt very much alone in the big city.

She was expecting me, since the hospital routinely asked the Visiting Nurse Service of New York to make a home visit to families who had been late in receiving prenatal care. This gave an opportunity for young families to learn about newborn care and how to find help when they needed it. I had visited many new mothers and their babies in their homes during the past year. In most

of the cases, I found the same problems. The major one was the feeling of isolation among the residents. Doors were kept bolted and very few people ventured into or out of the buildings. Yet, these young mothers had so much in common.

I asked Maria if she knew who in her neighborhood had new babies. She hadn't met anyone but was eager to make friends. As the visiting nurse in this community, I was a common link among these new mothers. During the next 2 weeks, I visited six new mothers in the area and invited each to attend a mother and baby coffee in Maria's apartment on Tuesday morning.

Two of the women agreed to come. Once they introduced themselves, their common interests around new babies allowed them to lower the barriers they had built up since moving to this new area. Although they would continue to face many problems in their future, the problem of isolation seemed to be overcome.

A visiting nurse is more than a link between residents and the health care system. This person can be a catalyst for neighbors finding solutions within their own walls. ■

Catherine Flynn Loveridge,
PhD, RN, PHN
1969

76

BRIAN

I arrived at my condo to find a children's birthday party in progress. Plates with partially eaten cake were on the table, and kids jubilantly swam in the pool. A few adults were sitting at the table. I found a chaise lounge and flopped on my stomach to read.

A minute after settling down I heard a loud thud. The gate to the pool clanged open and someone was screaming. I looked up to see a young woman picking up a young boy from the side of the pool's Jacuzzi. She was the one screaming. The little boy was limp. The woman was running around the perimeter of the pool, yelling for help. Suddenly the atmosphere became chaotic.

I got up from my chair thinking "Oh God he looks bad." The boy was pale, glassy-eyed, with a limp body. "What happened?" I asked.

"I don't know, he slipped and hit his head I think, I didn't see. He was floating" she replied.

I grabbed my towel and placed it on the cement and said, "Put him on the towel." Oh dear, I thought, I'm the only one here who knows what to do. A cardiac nurse more than 12 years, I felt frozen. I have 10 people staring at me and a hysterical mother. At work everyone acts as a team.

Sue Gemar Lloyd, RN
1997

I pointed at a woman. "You go call the paramedics." Then I decided to do the ABCs. OK, Let's see, airway is open—breathing, he's breathing, shallowly. Cardiac, he has a pulse around 100. He didn't respond to his name except to look in my direction. He started to vomit. His mother and I log-rolled him onto his side to maintain his airway. Then we put him in rescue position and waited. I'd been in a million code situations and I couldn't think of anything else to do but wait. The paramedics arrived quickly.

They questioned the mother. I then relayed what I knew. They quickly put him on oxygen, checked his vital signs, and started an IV. He was scooped up and off in a flash.

Everyone who had been around the pool had vanished after the ambulance arrived. I felt deserted and alone. Anticlimactic. I packed up my things and started home. As I walked, I could not help but ponder the timing of things.

Two months later I received a note in the mail. "Thank you so much for helping at the pool in July with my son. We are just so thankful that you knew what to do. It took me quite a while to find out who you were because we were invited to the birthday party and don't live in that complex. Just wanted you to know that Brian did OK after a day or so. He just started school, he is normal and healthy and doing just fine. Thank you. Diane (Brian's Mom)." ■

CHIEF

I was approached by the home care agency's administrative director to case manage and care for someone who happened to be a physician. The physician was a well-loved oncologist.

I was astonished to learn that the patient was Dr. Graham. I'd known him for nearly 15 years. As nurse, I had taken care of many of his patients. He was well-respected by many people, including myself. I could not say no to being his primary home care nurse.

As I arrived at his home my heart was pounding. As I approached Dr. Graham, he looked up at me and waved a hello. He couldn't speak because he had a permanent tracheostomy.

Dr. Graham had previously been diagnosed with kidney cancer and has been doing quite well. Now he was fighting metastatic renal cancer that had spread to his thyroid, lungs, and liver. I knew he would be a complex assignment. Besides having the trach, which required care twice a day and frequent suctioning, Dr. Graham had a central IV line, a feeding tube, injections for pain control, IV medications, blood transfusions, and chemotherapy. After my assessment, I knew he would require nursing visits twice a day.

In my car that day, sitting behind the wheel, I cried so hard that it hurt.

When I arrived the next day, I wondered how I should refer to the patient. Surely, calling him Dr. Graham would be too formal, and Randall would not be respectful. Because Dr. Graham was an administrator and chief of staff at a hospital, I asked him "Is it all right if I refer to you as 'Chief'?" He signaled OK.

I never leave a patient's home without asking "Is there anything else I can do for you?" It has always been important to me to communicate openly and honestly, as much as the patient and family desire, including discussing death and dying issues when appropriate. My holistic caring practice for patients is driven by empathy; I always put myself in the place of the patients, looking at what I would want in such a situation. It was always important for me to inquire how Mrs. Graham was doing, because she was the primary caregiver in the home. If she was too exhausted or not in good spirits, she could not be available for him.

The hardest thing for me to do was to discuss the Chief's knowledge of his prognosis. Discussing death and dying issues requires appropriate timing. I knew it was time for this discussion when the Chief experienced an episode of projectile bleeding from his trach—this occurred just as I was leaving from my second visit of the day.

He was frightened by the experience. After the situation was brought under control and considering the amount of blood loss, I suggested "Chief, I think you should go to the hospital." He wrote, "I don't want to go to the hospital." I clarified, "Do you want to remain at home?" "Yes, I want to be home no matter what." I moved closer to him. I said, "I am here for you—use me in any way required, and I will do whatever I can to make your wish of remaining in your home come true. I will also make sure you experience no suffering from pain." I assured him I would always be available for him. I kept my pager on 24 hours a day. "Are you afraid of dying?" I asked nervously. Chief wrote on his slate pad, "I am not afraid to die, only concerned with how it will happen." A warm smile appeared as I kissed his forehead, saying, "I will see that you are comfortable in your home."

Chief was friendly and kind. I remember him wanting his wife to get his lab coat for me during his trach bleeding episode. I assured him getting blood on my clothes was the least of my concerns—he was all that mattered.

Time became the one thing we didn't have. Chief became weaker and more dependent. It was more and more difficult to see him, but I had to remain strong. Chief's wishes were put in motion. I felt a deep spiritual connection, and wrote a special poem for Chief. He was able to read it before he lapsed into a coma. ∎

Rita Callahan, BSN, RN
1996

MARILYN

Marilyn was a woman in her late 30s who had been diagnosed about 3 months earlier with a widely metastatic cancer. Her first symptom had been a pathologic fracture of her shoulder, which occurred when she picked up a telephone to answer a call. She had a rapidly progressive course and was admitted a short time later for increasing shortness of breath. It soon became clear that she would die in the very near future.

My colleague asked her what was important to her. She replied that she had always hoped to be married, but she and her boyfriend kept putting off the date. With the help of a multitude of people, a wedding was hastily arranged for the next day. Her financial situation was dismal, so the license was obtained and paid for by a special patient fund we kept for emergencies. The hospital chaplain agreed to perform the ceremony. The photographer from the medical media department would take pictures. Flowers and a cake were brought in and a lovely white negligee was bought to serve as a wedding dress. Marilyn's mother and brother arrived from out of town. We draped a sheet over the equipment in the room so it would not look as much like a hospital environment.

The wedding was held around noon. Although in a terribly weakened condition, Marilyn was a very happy bride. She died about 4 hours later surrounded by her new husband and family.

For years I have been wearing a button on my lab coat: 'Oncology Nurses Say Never Postpone a Pleasure.' For me, it sums up a philosophy I have developed after nearly 2 decades in my field. I am constantly reminded to try to live each day as if it were my last and to not have any regrets about things I wished I had taken the time to enjoy. ∎

Cindy Jones, MS, RN, AOCN
1996

THE MARINOS

I have a strong recollection of the director of my LPN program calling me into her office and telling me that I would never make it as a nurse because I was 'too soft.' I entered the ranks of nursing with the impression that somehow my emotions were a liability and that I needed to learn to keep them in check. It was not until several years later that I discovered that my liability was indeed an asset.

After becoming a registered nurse, I began working in an oncology chemotherapy clinic. One of my first patients was Mrs. Marino. I found her in the waiting room and introduced myself. She, in turn, introduced me to her two daughters. They were extremely attentive to their mother and Mrs. Marino, somewhat reserved, let her daughters do much of the talking.

I escorted Mrs. Marino into a room to wait for her exam with the oncologist. As I was helping her tie the back of her gown, I could hear what sounded like sniffles and attempts to hide her tears. I sat down next to her and asked what was wrong. Much to the family's shock, her husband had just been told that he, too, had breast cancer. This extremely rare malignancy in men had struck out of the blue, and the family was now reeling from the news that both members of the couple now had to fight cancer. Mrs. Marino said that the girls were devastated, and yet they were trying desperately to hide their despondency from her. I listened and acknowledged Mrs. Marino's sadness, reassuring her that we would try our best to get her husband through his chemotherapy with as few complications as possible.

Upon meeting Mr. Marino, it was easy to see how much he and his wife loved each other, and how close their daughters were to both of them. As Mr. Marino's treatment evolved, the daughters slowly began talking to me about their fears, frustrations, and despair in thinking about the possibility of losing both their parents to cancer. They felt that it was unfair, and I agreed with them.

As I grew to know the family, I found myself absorbing more and more of the girls' sadness. It made me try to orchestrate their father's treatment regimen, such that his discomfort would be minimized, and his care would be highly customized to his needs. I always remembered which vein he preferred for his chemo. I knew he liked to lie on his left side with a pillow behind his back and between his knees since this decreased the pain in his lower spine. Orange juice was too acidic for his taste, so I had apple juice ready when he needed to take his pills.

As the treatment progressed, Mr. Marino appeared to be worsening. Nonetheless, his family continued to glow with reports of a slightly improved appetite and more time spent out on the patio. When he came in for treatment, he would wait until his wife and daughters went to lunch before telling me about how dependent he felt, and how much his illness had influenced the lives of his young daughters. This was not a good way to die, he told me, and he wanted it to be over so that he would not have to burden them anymore. I listened attentively and acknowledged his despair. But I also told him that I thought his daughters were giving back to him for all he had done in their lives. They knew he would indeed be there for them if they were sick and so now they wanted to be present for him.

The following Monday I was told that Mr. Marino had been hospitalized over the weekend. He was not doing well. I walked over to the inpatient unit, and as I rounded the corner, I saw the three women sobbing in the hallway outside Mr. Marino's room. "Oh no," I thought, "He died. I'm not ready to handle this, and I don't know what to say to his wife and daughters." Without realizing what I was doing, I turned around to go back into the clinic, telling myself I had to check on something from the pharmacy. I needed an excuse to escape. Tears were starting to run from my eyes, and I felt myself losing control. How could I comfort the family if I was in such a state myself? Then I told myself, "Your tears are not the issue here. Their comfort is." I turned and went back down the hallway. Upon seeing the family, my tears began to flow again, but I continued toward the three women. The daughters saw me first, called my name, and fell into my arms. We cried and sobbed together and comforted one another.

I cried again at Mr. Marino's wake and apologized to Mrs. Marino and her daughters. I told them that I felt guilty for needing comfort myself when it was their father and husband whom they were mourning. "No, no, Debi," the girls said, "Don't apologize for that. You have no idea how it made us feel, seeing you cry for our dad. We know how much you liked him and what good care you took of him. It's so comforting to us to know that he meant that much to you too." I have been through more than 20 years of cancer nursing, and I still have that 'emotional problem.' Tears can exemplify the special connections we feel with our patients and their families—some of whom are hard to forget. ∎

Deborah Boyle, MSN, RN, AOCN
1998

82

MRS. SIMPSON

Just graduated from a baccalaureate nursing program, I was armed with many ideas, but few practical applications of the theory that I had learned. I was assigned to a 52-year-old woman on a general psychiatric unit. She was severely depressed. Mrs. Simpson could not care for herself. Her lack of self-care and subsequent loss of weight and stamina showed this. She had minimal support in the community. The psychiatric unit staff took on the primary caregiving role.

One weekend afternoon, Mrs. Simpson was agitated and screaming, and not responding to our calm support. Initially, I thought she was having a reaction to the medication we were giving for her depression. I administered medication to counteract these reactions, but it was not effective in calming Mrs. Simpson. I moved her to a private room and decreased the stimulation around her by dimming lights and decreasing the noise from the hallways. Since there were no other medication orders, I called the attending physician. He was concerned about her lack of response to the medication. He suggested that we try 'wet packs' to calm Mrs. Simpson.

Luc R. Pelletier, MSN, RN, CS, CPHQ
1980

"Wet packs?" I had read about this treatment, used in the early 1900s, but had never observed or administered the treatment. I asked one of the other nurses on the unit that day about wet packs and what to do. "Come here, I'll show you" was her response. "The experience of wet packs is like running into a cold ocean, diving in, and coming out to be wrapped in a warm towel or blanket—it's very soothing," she said. I indeed had experienced this and always felt calm after wrapping myself warmly.

We let Mrs. Simpson know that we would treat her with 'wet packs' and that this would help to calm her. We prepared buckets of ice and placed Mrs. Simpson on a stretcher in the middle of the room. We wrapped her in sheets. We then dumped ice and ice water onto the sheets. Mrs. Simpson was startled but we talked her through the procedure. We then wrapped her in wool blankets, swaddling her like a mummy. This calmed her considerably. The screaming stopped almost immediately and her agitation seemed to leave.

I stayed with her throughout the procedure. We were left alone after the wrapping. I stroked her forehead and hair and told her I would stay with her until she felt better. She eventually fell asleep.

Mrs. Simpson eventually responded to the antidepressant medication. She slowly began to care for herself and looked forward to returning home. ∎

EDNA

My husband and I and our 4-year-old had just moved to California. We were renting a small house near the university and were just beginning to settle into the neighborhood. On one side of our house lived a young family with three children; on the other side, a retired couple named Edna and Tom. We had introduced ourselves when my son was out playing in the front yard and had a brief conversation in which I stated that I was a nurse and would be teaching at the university.

We were about to celebrate our first Thanksgiving in California. As a young nurse, I never minded working Christmas in the hospital so that the married staff could be home with their children as long as I could have Thanksgiving with my family. When I moved away to attend graduate school and later married while in Colorado, my husband and I created a new 'family' of friends who joined us for the annual Thanksgiving dinner. This year would be our first without either our 'old' or 'new' family.

I suppose I was feeling a bit sorry for myself when the phone rang. It was Edna and she sounded upset. Would I please come over to her house right away? "Of course," I said. While my husband watched

our son, I dashed next door and heard Edna call through the screen door for me to come in and come into her bedroom. There was Edna, sitting at the edge of the bed in a loose nightgown with large bandages covering her chest and a box of 4-by-4 bandages on the nightstand. "Cathy, I hardly know you, but you're a nurse and so I called you. I came home last night from the hospital. I went in last Wednesday and they did a mastectomy for cancer. Tom is so upset that he can't help me right now. I'm supposed to change my dressing and I don't know where to start. My daughter and her family are bringing dinner here this afternoon and I don't want her to see me like this."

At that moment, she started to cry. I sat down on the chair opposite her and spoke softly. "Edna, when I was a visiting nurse in Boston, I used to change dressings like this all the time. Let's see what they sent home with you and figure out where we go from here." As I began to take stock of the supplies in the box, I realized that there wasn't a sufficient supply to last until her next doctor's appointment. "Let's make a list of what you will need until Monday and I'll pick them up at the pharmacy in the shopping center. They're open until noon today. While I'm gone, I want you to choose what you want to wear for Thanksgiving dinner." I then left for the store.

While I was driving away from the house, I began to think about how, by virtue of my profession, my neighbor recognized me immediately as someone who could be trusted to know what to do. Her confidence in me helped me to put aside my own self absorption and focus on what was really important.

I returned with boxes of large dressings and enough supplies to last over the weekend. As I removed the old dressing, Edna talked about how scared she was when she learned she had cancer, but that her doctor was confident she had caught it in the early stages. She had not talked about her surgery with anyone because she didn't want to worry her family.

As I applied the new dressings, I could see Edna begin to relax and later to talk about her grandchildren who would be coming over for dinner. I helped Edna finish getting dressed and I realized that our friendship had moved to a new level. I would be there as a neighbor and friend, but also as a nurse. ∎

Catherine Flynn Loveridge,
PhD, RN, PHN
1983

LALU OF INDIA

The people of the village knew that I was a nurse practitioner in the United States. I had come with my husband to give continued support to the clinic that we opened in 1989 in a village in southern India. I wasn't able to speak the native tongue of the people of this village, but somehow they didn't seem to mind. I did what I could to assist the physician and help the people in ways that didn't need words.

One morning I was sitting among the people as my husband conversed with them and found out how things were going. There was a mother in the crowd of people who had a sick child on her lap. Many of her relatives were sitting close by and everyone seemed to take their turn comforting the child, but to no avail. I reached out my hands to the mother in a gesture that was asking if I could hold the child. She handed me Lalu. I then motioned to have her sit next to me so that her 7-month-old son could keep his eyes on her and wouldn't be frightened that I was holding him.

As I began to slowly rock little Lalu, I did Reiki, a form of ancient energy healing. I just gently put my arms around little Lalu as he sat on my lap and asked God and the universe to bless him. Everyone watched me. I then began to sing a song to this little fellow because I learned from my own children how comforting music can be. It was no more than 5 minutes when I noticed Lalu's head began to droop. Finally he was falling asleep—something he hadn't been able to do well since his fever began 24 hours previously. I continued to hold him and after he was in a deep sleep, gave him back to his mother. Her smile was beautiful and her eyes spoke beams of gratitude. The crowd became quiet. They were amazed! They asked my husband "What did your wife from America do?" He said "Loved Lalu and rocked him to sleep."

We were reminded how love needs no words and transcends any barriers of language and culture. When Lalu awakened, he had no fever and was back to his playful, energetic 7-month-old delight. ∎

Mary Kodiath, MS, RNC, ANP
1997

CINDY AND STEVEN

I had just returned from an exciting presentation on how newborns could be comforted by sounds similar to those they had heard in the uterus. The speaker gave examples of infants who would become quiet and listen intently to the sounds of Mozart, a recording of a heartbeat, or to water sounds. These sounds were initially introduced to the growing fetus in its warm uterine home by the mother. This is done either through her normal daily activities of living or through the placement of a tape recorder on her gravid abdomen. Once infants are born, they seem to listen and recognize these sounds once again.

Little did I realize that I could put this newfound knowledge to use so quickly. As a clinical nurse specialist in a labor and delivery unit, I was often asked to see patients who were experiencing some difficulty in their birthing experience. That morning, I was asked by the nursing staff to visit with Cindy and Steven, a young couple who were having their first baby. Cindy had labored much of the night and was nearly exhausted. Steven didn't appear to have had much sleep either, and the nurses reported that he had faithfully stayed at Cindy's side all night, helping her to find a comfortable position or 'breathe' through the contractions. Progress had been made and Cindy's cervix had dilated to 8 centimeters, yet the couple was frantic—Cindy was sobbing, and Steven was in tears. Apparently, the baby's heart rate had risen consistently over the last 2 hours, and the heart rate pattern was suggestive of impending fetal distress. Cindy's blood pressure also had risen to a level of concern. The doctor had just informed them that the baby would need to be delivered by Cesarean section if things didn't change soon.

After assessing Cindy's and the baby's condition, I pulled up a chair beside her bed. "Well, tell me now, what is going on?" I asked. The young couple could hardly talk through the sobs and tears. Cindy related her very realistic fears about the possibility of a Cesarean delivery. She was exhausted, afraid of the unknown, and clearly uncomfortable. "I just wish there was something I could do," Steven said. "A father's role is to protect, and I can't do anything but sit here and watch helplessly."

Suddenly, I was inspired to try some of the concepts introduced at the conference. "Certainly, they wouldn't cause any harm," I thought, "and they might actually help."

After I had positioned Cindy again to make her comfortable and assigned Steven the job of wiping her brow with a cool cloth, I related to them the concepts about quieting techniques that I'd learned at the conference. If they would work on newborns, maybe they would work on the 'about-to-be-born' infant. I asked Steven if they ever played music or talked to the baby. A big smile appeared on his face and he said, "I put my face on Cindy's big tummy and sing to the baby all the time."

"How does the baby respond?" I asked.

Cindy said that the baby would either become quiet after being fairly active or would begin to kick and move about. They were both eager to try 'quieting.' Maybe the baby was as exhausted, afraid, and uncomfortable as they were.

Steven began singing the sweet songs to his baby that he'd been singing every evening over the last few months. At first there was increased movement inside that tightly drawn abdomen. Could the baby have been turning toward the sounds that she or he had so often heard? I could hardly believe my eyes as I watched the fetal heart rate pattern on the monitor begin to slow to a more normal level. There was even more variability in the heart rate, and that was a very reassuring sign. Steven talked to the baby: "I am right here little one. Mommy and Daddy can hardly wait to see you. We love you. You are going to be all right." Sounds of reassurance and complete love.

Cindy quickly dilated to 9 centimeters and felt the urge to push. The physician, who had also witnessed the change on the fetal monitor at the nurse's station, quickly returned to the room and was surprised to see Steven gently singing to Cindy's swollen abdomen. Properly positioned to push and with Steven still singing and talking to the baby, it was safely delivered vaginally.

Who is to know what really happened in this story? Did the reassuring sounds that had become so familiar over the last few months comfort the baby? Did Steven's soft whispers of love comfort Cindy and also have a positive physiological effect on her and the baby? Maybe hope was restored in a seemingly hopeless situation. Whatever the explanation, the effect was the same: the bond of human love between mother, father, and baby was reinforced with the simple sound of Steven's voice.

The process of a couple working together to comfort and soothe one another and the little life within creates a beautiful bond that is necessary to nurture and grow new life.

I often reflect on this experience. It was helpful not only to Cindy, Steven, and baby Andrew, but it was also meaningful to me to see the evidence of faith, hope, and love. ∎

Jaynelle F. Stichler, DNSc, RN
1986

THE OLD TEXAN

Early in my nursing career, I was working the day shift and had been pulled from the adolescent psychiatric unit to the oncology unit. I was assigned to 10 or 11 patients for nursing care.

The work that morning had been fast and furious. About 11 am, I was covering all the patients. I was answering lights, providing care, rushed, and moving fast. That's when the light went on in the last room at the end of the hall. It was a single room and I did not know the patient.

I walked into the room and saw an old woman sitting up in bed. I greeted her and asked her what she needed. She replied in a very thick Texas accent, "I need the bedpan!" I said "OK" and started looking for her bedpan. She quickly replied, "Are you going to do it?" I said that there was no one else to do it. She replied "I don't want you to do it; I want the bedpan." I explained that I was the only one who could help her. And again, but louder, she said "I don't want you to do it; I want the bedpan."

I decided to use a different tactic and told her that she really only had one other option, and I was sure she wouldn't want me to have

to come back and change her bed. I was convinced this approach would work, even though I was calling her bluff. She looked me straight in the eye with the conviction of a rattlesnake and said "I don't want you to do it; I want the bedpan."

Her determination and anxiety as well as mine increased by the second. She began repeating in her very convincing Texas accent, "I want the bedpan; I want the bedpan." In the midst of the hurricane of words I thought, "Why is she doing this?" Then, it came to me. She was afraid I would see her!

Between "I want the bedpan" and "I don't want you to do it," I said "Ma'am, why don't you lift up your back end; I will place the bedpan under you. You keep the covers on and I won't look, I promise." She was on the end of ". . . the bedpan" and stopped cold. She looked at me, lifted her back end up, and used the bedpan—the whole time keeping her privacy and dignity.

When she was finished, she said "You're not so bad for a male nurse!" For the rest of the shift, whenever she had to use the bedpan she requested the 'male nurse' to help her!

Sometimes nurses have to stop, look, and listen, and the answer will become clear. The old Texan was determined not to lose what was important to her: privacy and dignity. I not only did not take those things from her, but left her with something else, respect. She left me something as well, as a permanent reminder. ∎

Rick Zoucha, DNSc, RN, CS
1982

DOM

It came as no surprise that I was assigned to work the night shift over Christmas my first year out of nursing school. When I arrived at work Christmas night, all was quiet, the lights were turned down, and the patients all appeared to be asleep.

One of my patients that night was Dom, a 51-year-old husband and father of three who was dying of cancer. We all knew the diagnosis and prognosis, at least intellectually. In the first 6 weeks of Dom's recovery from a CABG, he started to have difficulty swallowing, and he lost 20 pounds. The same surgeon who had performed Dom's CABG opened him back up to discover a massive, inoperable esophageal tumor. He came to our unit postoperatively, as he had following his previous surgery. I don't remember why he stayed with us, other than that our caseload was slow, and could give him lots of attention.

During report I was told that Dom's wife, his two teenage daughters, and son had spent the day with him. They had opened presents, and Dom had even managed to eat a few bites of food that they had brought from home. His vital signs were stable, but he was worn out from his busy day. I peeked in on Dom as I started my shift. He was asleep, so I began with my other patient.

Just as I returned to the desk, Dom's call light came on. He needed help standing to void. I helped him stand and stood behind the curtain (he wanted some privacy and we all tried to provide what we could). When he was finished, we started talking as I went through my routine assessment. He asked me about my holiday, and he told me about his visit with his family. Everyone had made it: his wife, the kids, even his brother had come in from out-of-state. We talked about the presents we both had given as well as received, and we talked of past Christmases. As I was settling him in to sleep, he asked me the time. "It's 11:30" I said. "Still Christmas?" he asked. "Yes." I turned the lights down and left as he closed his eyes.

The quiet of the night continued, until about 2:00 am. I heard the thud of plastic hitting the floor. The sound had come from Dom's room. I rushed in to find Dom standing at the side of the bed. The urinal, half full, had hit the floor.

"Why did you get up without me?" I asked. He had never done that before. He just shook his head and apologized. Then I noticed that his pajama pants were soaked with urine, as was his bed. I helped him into the chair and went about changing the sheets and getting Dom clean and dry. He was not very talkative and sat unusually quietly as I went about my tasks.

I helped Dom to bed and tucked him in. I medicated him for his pain. "What time is it?" he asked, once again. "It's 2:15" I said. "What day?" "It's December 26, the day after Christmas." "Good" he replied. Then he asked something that he had never before requested. "Stay with me, Barb. Please just sit with me." I pulled up a chair, lowered the siderail, and took his hand. He squeezed it tight. "Thank you."

We said very little, and soon Dom closed his eyes, as if to sleep. I noticed that his breathing was starting to get slightly labored and irregular. A coworker looked in on us and mouthed, "Are you OK?" I mouthed back, "Call his family." I knew that Dom had waited for Christmas to be over to die. His heart rate slowly dropped on the monitor. When the coworker returned to turn off the alarm, Dom, startled, opened his eyes, looked at me, and again asked the time and day. I whispered, "Christmas is over, Dom." He smiled, squeezed my hand tightly and closed his eyes. His breathing once again became irregular. At 2:30 am, December 26, 1978, Dom, husband of Phyllis, father of Dom Jr., Elizabeth and Theresa, took his last breath, as I sat and held his hand. ∎

Barb McGurgan, MSN, RN, CCRN
1978

INDIAN AND ALASKAN WOMEN

More than 500 American Indian, Alaskan, and Canadian native women gathered in Portland, Oregon. At a health fair staffed by volunteer RNs, 130 women lined up waiting for a chance to experience therapeutic touch (TT).

The health fair offered many booths—however, most of the attendees were gathered at the Touch Booth. Before long, the women changed from asking if they could "see what this touch is," to requesting "a healing."

Soon four elders, in traditional dress, came for their 'treatments.' One, appearing to look deep within my soul with her warm and wise brown eyes said to me, "You have good hands." She then gathered the three other grandmothers to sit between the two booths on folding chairs, an act endorsing the activities of both the Touch Booth and the Breast Health Booth. Seventy-five women were screened for breast cancer. Most had never had a previous clinical breast examination. None had ever seen or heard of TT as taught by nurses. Others did know

the way of the healer and were pleased the healers were present to offer their gifts.

When women gather together to help women, a safe environment is created. Their sisters nurture them, offer them support, and healing occurs. The nurses who offered their touch to help and to heal, set the stage for many healing encounters to occur throughout the conference week. As the week proceeded, participants asked "Are the healers returning?" On the last conference day, two nurse practitioners set up tables in the gathering hall to do touch therapies. Many inquired if it was too late for their clinical breast check and mammogram. More health teaching was performed.

This group of nurses had entered the world of Indian women through the opened door of hands-on touch therapy. Through the trust established, they delivered a necessary clinical screening. During the fair, three women were found to have suspicious lesions for breast cancer and were referred for immediate medical intervention. Many of the women stated, "I never would have had this exam at home."

The volunteer nurses who offered their hands and hearts all had a profound personal experience during this event. When asked to describe the event, they all brought the same look to the soft glaze of their eyes, reflecting something beyond experience. . .a wonder. . .a knowing. . .a deep gratitude to life. By offering healing to others, they attained a profound healing of their own. ∎

Rosze Barrington, MS, RN, ANP, CS
1996

MARTY

I had noticed the blond teenager strewn across the couch in the waiting room each time I went to call in the next patient. The boy looked flushed, thin, and ill. I was pretty new at my role as a nurse practitioner and at my job as an AIDS research nurse. AZT was also new. Many patients wanted to enroll in this very first AZT clinical trial. I was expecting a new patient that morning, a 30-year-old man recently recovering from PCP pneumonia. I was surprised when a middle-aged man approached me and asked brusquely, "When is someone going to see my son? He's been waiting here for over an hour." His son, who looked 17, was my new patient. Over the course of the next year, I got to know Marty very well. He taught me a great deal about the healing power of being a nurse.

With AIDS, you can be terribly ill with an opportunistic infection one minute and then feel better and go forward with the knowledge that the bottom could fall out again at any moment. In 1986, AIDS was a death sentence.

Marty was an accomplished artist. His neo-impressionistic paintings and sculptures were becoming nationally recognized. He had one-man shows on the east and west coasts. He had a studio, an agent, and a gallery operator. He had no energy. He was frightened. Marty explained, "As soon as I walk into a room I start looking for a place to sit down. I start worrying if anyone will notice that I look too thin." He hadn't expected to get AIDS.

I knew enough about life, illness, and dying to understand that the task of nursing is to help the individual realize his deepest inner resources in order to cope with his crisis. Marty's parents were always there for him. His dad, Steve, always said "You have to play the hand you're dealt." Muriel, Marty's mom, was a retired RN and baccalaureate professor.

Marty helped me understand how to create a therapeutic relationship beyond the bounds of what bedside nursing had taught me. Suddenly I was the primary care provider, the physical, mental, emotional, and spiritual advisor to people my own age dying of AIDS. Now, once I met a patient, I would see him regularly for the next few months or years of his life.

Marty took to me like a life preserver in a storm. He was needy, vulnerable, and honest, and I was his nurse. He called when he needed to talk. He confided his fears, his desires, and his disappointments. He sought comfort and encouragement. He wanted consistency from me. There was no space for backing away. He and all my other patients needed me to be steadfast.

The experience with Marty and others in the AIDS Research Center forced me to grow and expand my emotional and psychological capacities at breakneck speed. I was becoming a more mature, experienced therapist and clinician with every patient visit. Integrating my professional and personal growth was a consuming responsibility.

Marty was handsome, talented, and an all-around attractive person. He was hard not to like. I had to adjust many of the boundaries I had set up around my patient–nurse relationship. My patients suddenly felt too much like friends, and I was constantly trying to learn detachment and balance.

Marty had seizures near the end and was unresponsive for more than 24 hours in the hospital. Though he still had paint spots on his hands and arms from his work, he now was absent. His body seemed vacant. I reached out and held his hand as I sat next to the bed. I started telling him how much I had learned from him, how much I cared about him, and how greatly I admired him. I was crying. I was looking at his hand in my hand, with the blue paint on the fingernail, and I said "I'll miss you." I let out a sob when he responded, "I'll miss you too." ∎

Joanne Santangelo, MSN, RN
1987

MILDRED
AND BUDDY

I have been a psychiatric nurse for close to 45 years, many of those years in an outpatient day-hospital program for patients with severe and persistent mental illness. Caring for the whole person presents challenges and lessons never taught in nursing school. Mildred, an 80-year-old patient, required admission to the hospital after a fall.

I went to see her and asked who was going to take care of her dog, Buddy, while she was there. "I don't have anyone except my neighbor and he is out of town." After giving it some thought, I called her home health nurse, who said she had gone by the patient's house but couldn't get in because Mildred had lost her house keys. She later went back and climbed in through a front window (standing on the trash can in order to reach high enough). She fed the dog but said she would be unable to continue to care for him. I called the Humane Society but they were unable to provide a foster home because Buddy would have to be put up for adoption after 2 weeks.

So I went to Mildred's home myself. I, too, stepped on the trash can, climbed in through the window, fed the dog, and took him

for a walk. He was delighted with the attention. I also discovered a group of feral cats living in her overgrown back yard. Several were quite young and ill.

The next day I made a return trip through the window and then out the back door. I managed to catch two of the cats (and was rather badly scratched in the process). Off we went to the emergency animal hospital for examination and subsequent euthanasia. I realized I could not go to the home every day, so I called my veterinarian and he agreed to board the dog until I could make further arrangements. (My cat would not approve of Buddy in our small apartment.) The vet gave Buddy a rabies shot (he had never had one), a bath, and a flea treatment which he badly needed, and finally agreed to do all this for free.

A friend from work has a yard and 4 dogs so he agreed to board Buddy for several weeks. I drove to the vet, got Buddy, and came back to the hospital to make the transfer. Buddy sat on my lap and licked me all the way. I got him out of the car and my friend came up behind us and leaned down. Buddy didn't see him coming and responded to the surprise by accidentally biting me and taking a piece out of my arm. My friend got the dog in his car and I went to the emergency room.

Three hours later I had been sewn up (about 10 stitches) and went back to work, only to receive a phone call from my friend saying that his dogs hated Buddy. In the nick of time another friend with a yard and a dog offered to take him. So Buddy was transported there, where he spent the next 3 weeks.

I continued to crawl through the patient's window nearly every day in order to feed the remaining cats in the backyard, all the while hoping the police would not see me breaking into the house. During this time Mildred's gas and electricity were cut off so everything in her refrigerator went bad. I received a bill from the ED and my insurance company wanted the name of the dog's owner, her attorney's name, and the name of her insurance company. I had not told Mildred about the bite and I refused to give the information, so I ended up paying the ED bill myself. Then my friend mentioned the cost of feeding Buddy, so I bought dog food and treats for him.

I visited Mildred at the rehab hospital, and she was very glad to know that Buddy was being cared for. "I miss him so much," she repeated at each visit. On the day she was finally going home, she looked in her purse and discovered she had her house keys after all.

All my window climbing had been unnecessary, but it did increase my agility. Mildred went home, Buddy went home, my stitches were removed, and all ended well—except my boss said, "Never do that stuff again, Gale". ∎

Gale Osborn, MA, RN, C
1996

SANDY

After my junior year in a baccalaureate nursing program, I was working as an LPN on an obstetrics unit at a local Catholic hospital. Each day began with shift report and morning rounds. Rounds consisted of checking each patient's vital signs, fluid output, and assessing postpartum bleeding.

One morning I entered Sandy's room and introduced myself to a pretty young woman with long blond hair. She burst into tears and cried for several minutes. Then she explained what was troubling her. She had delivered a baby boy the night before, but gave up the baby for adoption because she was an unwed mother. She was unable to support the baby financially on her own. She felt ashamed because she was Catholic and unmarried and had had a baby out of wedlock. She cried as she spoke of her love for her baby—a baby she had not even seen, and she wondered if this was the best way to give him up.

She continued to cry. I was struck by her sadness, gentleness, and how alone she seemed with her pain. She was also in a room by herself and added that she didn't expect any visitors during her stay. We talked a bit more and I promised to return when I had completed my rounds.

Later I told her I had seen her baby and described him to her. We talked about the possibility of her actually seeing him. We realized that this would make the baby more real and the loss much more real. We also realized that it could help with the grieving and mourning that would follow.

I arranged for her to see her baby at the nursery. We walked together from her room at the end of the west wing to the nursery in the south wing. She cried as she looked at her baby through the nursery window. We walked back to her room, where she continued to sob. She spoke about her baby, how he had looked, and how hard this was to do. She felt she was doing the best thing for him but her pain was enormous. I listened to her and hugged her as she cried.

I never saw her or her baby again. I was off for the next few days. I was told the baby left with the adoption agency and the mother had gone home.

I am glad I was able to listen to her needs and be sensitive to her loss. It has been more than 20 years since this happened, and it brings tears to my eyes as I recall her pain and the enormity of her loss. I am glad I could be there. ∎

Jane Milazzo, MS, RN, LPN, CS
1982

BETSY

Snow was falling gently as I walked the short distance to the hospital. I was a senior student nurse working the night shift in pediatrics. It would have been my day off, but the unit was short staffed and the pay for working on my day off would help me buy a new pair of shoes for Christmas.

The ward was quiet, but a heartbreaking story unfolded. Betsy, age 5, and her 2½-year-old brother had been found earlier that day. Both were dressed in shorts, in a house with no heat, and very little food. The little boy had pneumonia, and Betsy had been taking care of him and would not leave his side. The mother frequently left them alone while she was working as a prostitute. Neighbors had discovered the children alone and called the police.

As I made my rounds I walked into their room. Betsy wakened easily while I was checking her brother's vital signs. "Is he going to be okay? I tried to help him get well." I assured her he was better and he would get well. She was such a beautiful little girl who had

taken on so much responsibility in her young life. I told her my name and that I would be there all night.

Later as I checked in on the two children, Betsy was awake. She smiled at me, said she felt good, and it was nice to be warm. Then tears fell from her eyes. I hugged her and we talked. She said her mother told her she would not get a doll for Christmas because she was a bad girl; then she looked up at me with tear-filled eyes and asked "Do you think I will get a doll from Santa?" I told her she would and that she had been a very good girl to take such good care of her brother. "My brother should get a present too" she said and I told her he would. She laid her head on her pillow and was soon asleep. Tears filled my eyes and I planned my shopping trip the next day.

Word got around quickly. Staff brought used and new clothing, toys, and even a little Christmas tree for the room.

Christmas Eve came and so did Santa, with a doll for Betsy and presents for her brother. Seeing a little girl hugging her new doll and knowing she and her brother were on their way to a foster home, and hopefully a better life, made it a wonderful Christmas and my old shoes were so comfortable! ∎

Patricia Robinson, BSN, RN
1958

PATTY

Patty was admitted to the ICU in respiratory distress, expectorating bright red blood from her lungs. Her diagnosis was unknown and she was placed on a ventilator. She had been having cold-like symptoms for 2 weeks. This illness in a seemingly robust 21-year-old woman was a shock to her and her family.

Patty was gravely ill. She required suctioning every 10 to 15 minutes, along with a series of diagnostic tests. I was her primary care nurse. Several physicians were consulted and a diagnosis of Goodpasture's syndrome was not made for about 48 hours. This is a rare disease of sudden onset causing combined lung and kidney failure.

Visiting hours were very restricted. The family was only allowed to visit her for 5 or 10 minutes, twice a day. Patty was critically ill and yet she maintained consciousness and was alert and oriented. Even though she became ill so quickly, she possessed a calm attitude and just wanted to spend as much time as possible with her husband to discuss what needed to happen if she died. She seemed to have an intuitive knowledge of her impending death.

Patty was in a cubicle next to the wall, and when the curtain was drawn, she was out of sight of the nurses' station. Our head nurse enforced the rigid visiting hours, yet I felt this couple needed to spend time together. Her husband was very helpful and not in the way of her care, although she was receiving frequent transfusions and ventilator care. I made the decision to violate the visiting rules, and let him sit on the side of the bed.

During these times, I would help them communicate. They discussed things like remarriage if she died, and care of their child, and how much they loved each other. I also spent time with her parents and allowed them to spend time with her.

On her third hospital day, she was taken to the operating room for bilateral nephrectomy. However, she died just prior to the procedure.

After her death, the family came to the ICU to see us and to thank us for all we had done. Her husband visited us several weeks later and expressed his gratitude for the priceless time he had spent with her.

Because we modified the rules, this family was able to face this tragic incident and deal with many issues that helped their grief process. I was so sad when she died—but I felt a sense of spiritual achievement in knowing that my decision was the right thing to do. I have been gratified by the relaxation of ICU visiting hours in recent years. ∎

Martha L. Scott, MSN, RN
1977

99

PAUL

It was late morning and I was getting ready to do an 'add on' case in the operating room where I worked as a certified registered nurse anesthetist.

Paul was 47 years old and had recently experienced an acute myocardial infarction. He had needed the intra-aortic balloon pump in the stages immediately following his heart attack. He was noticeably nervous about his impending surgery and was eager to talk to someone.

As I started his IV, I tried to distract him from his preoccupation with the upcoming procedure. We talked about his family and, most notably, his 13-year-old daughter of whom he was very proud. The operating room nurse informed me that they were ready for me to bring Paul into the operating room.

The operation began and Paul was eager to continue talking. He opened up to me about his life, his fears regarding his recent illness, and the love he felt for his family. What had on the surface previously appeared as a straightforward, hour-long procedure was now progressing into more complex surgery that extended well into its second hour. Paul's anxiety grew as time passed, despite the anesthetic drugs. Due to

Kathleen Hanna, EdD, RN, CRNA
1986

his cardiac history, the surgeon did not want him over-sedated during the procedure, so I tried to manage the fine line between sedation and general anesthesia.

The operation continued, complications arose, and Paul began to lose blood. We began to hang blood and increase his IV fluids but, despite our efforts, he began to show hemodynamic instability. His physical condition deteriorated rapidly, accompanied by profuse ST changes on his ECG. His heart damage steadily increased. Paul was still awake but realized things were not progressing as smoothly as we all had anticipated. It became apparent that the anesthesiologist and I would need to put him to sleep and control his airway through intubation.

I explained the situation to Paul, and I could see the intense fear in his eyes. I held his hand and tried to reassure him before administering anesthesia and placing the endotracheal tube down his throat. Right before he lost consciousness he said, "Please tell my family I love them." I told him I would and that I would go to visit them. Paul never woke up. He continued to deteriorate and had another massive myocardial infarction with cardiac arrest from which he could not be resuscitated.

I went to his family after the surgeon had spoken with them and gave them Paul's message. These were the last words he said—his final thought. The family said it gave them some comfort, and I was glad to be able to deliver it to them. ∎

KATHY

I feel very lucky to have chosen nursing as a profession. During the almost 30 years of my career, I have been a primary nurse in GYN oncology, a home health nurse, an OB nurse and manager, university instructor, entrepreneur, and hospital administrator. I have always been amazed at the level of trust that patients and their families have placed in their nurse, a virtual stranger.

I was a fairly new OB nurse manager in a large East coast university hospital. I had just completed some requisite paperwork and decided to make rounds. First stop was the nursery where I volunteered to bathe or feed a newborn. There's nothing like holding a little bundle of new life, feeling little wiggle movements and observing facial expressions: instant stress reduction! Then, on to visit the moms.

It was dusk when I knocked and entered one of our few private rooms. Seated in the dark, alone, was a woman with her head down and shoulders collapsed into her chest, softly crying. I introduced myself and sat down to talk with her. In a very quiet voice Kathy explained that she had just

delivered her first child, a boy, prematurely and was absolutely terrified. The newborn was in the NICU and she hadn't yet been there to visit him. Her husband had visited the newborn but now was home getting some sleep.

I asked her if she'd like me to take her to visit her son. After checking with the NICU nurses to be sure it was a good time to visit, I brought her to the unit in a wheelchair. I explained what she could expect to see as we waited for the elevator. Entering a busy, crowded NICU is intimidating, and more so at wheelchair eye level when the newborn is yours.

Kathy spent time visiting her son, touching and speaking softly to him as his nurse told her about his condition, reassuring her that he would be just fine. After a while, I brought her back to her room and got her settled in for the evening.

I can recall this event in such stunning detail because for the past 12 years I have received a Christmas card from Kathy reminding me of that evening. She always lets me know how active and bright Ryan is and there's always a recent photo of Ryan.

What is amazing to me is that Kathy always takes the time to find out where I am. I've had three career moves since that night, moving in and out of state twice.

Kathy's effort to write to me every year for the past 12 years is incredibly heartwarming. After all, what I did was nothing that special. It was all in a day's work of a nurse. ∎

Deborah Dunne, MSN, RN, MBA
1986

LISA

Several years ago, I was running a pilot research project in which I was interviewing ventilator-dependent patients. Some of my colleagues questioned the feasibility of such a project. But I was determined and was motivated to treat ventilator-dependent patients as any other patients. I was notified of a young woman who was willing to have me visit her in her home and who might be willing to participate in the study. This young woman, Lisa, was in her mid-30s and had ALS. The only body function she had remaining was the ability to blink her eyes.

As I stepped onto Lisa's front porch, I momentarily paused and questioned whether I would be able to carry out the project in a manner that would be respectful of patients and still be sound research. My hesitation dissipated as I responded to the warm, relaxed environment that permeated Lisa's home. I was shown into the dining room that had been converted into a bedroom. Lisa's mother and father spent each day with her, along with a sitter who tended to her physical needs.

When I first saw Lisa, I was overwhelmed with the vibrant personality reflected in her eyes. I had worried that I would feel sympathy for her, but instead I immediately felt a unique closeness

with her. She was thin and pale, with her light brown hair pulled back from her face. The position of her trunk, arms and legs was obviously that of someone who has been posed because of lack of voluntary movement. Yet there was no doubt of the energy and strength that exuded from Lisa.

I pulled a chair to the side of the bed and sat facing her. I explained the project and asked her if she would be willing to participate. We worked out a code using her blinking. Most of the questions I had to ask her were on a Likert scale so I made a sign that had all of the possible answers. She blinked when I pointed to the answer that she preferred. After just a few questions, I perceived that it was uncomfortable for her to keep looking down at me, so I asked if she would mind if I sat on the bed. That way our eyes were level and we both seemed more relaxed.

The specific moment I will always remember is when I asked her a question about how involved she wanted to be in decisions about her care. When she blinked her eyes at the 'very involved' option, the blink was much more forceful than I had seen at any other question and I began to laugh. I said, "Well, that was certainly an emphatic answer!" Her eyes twinkled and I could sense her struggle to smile, apparent only by the slight upward turn of the corner of her eyes. At that moment I felt a closeness with her that I have rarely felt with any other patient. She relaxed noticeably, and I felt we were communicating on a level beyond blinking.

Lisa kept going until all the questions were answered. While Lisa rested, I talked with her parents in the kitchen. They commented on the comfort level Lisa and I had been able to achieve so quickly. It was a mutual admiration session because I applauded them for their commitment to her and for the wonderful atmosphere they had maintained in the home. They confided in me how difficult it was for them sometimes to see her this way and how their lives had changed since Lisa had become bedridden. They did not feel they were doing anything special, but they thanked me for the personal manner with which I treated Lisa.

On my way out, I thanked Lisa for participating in the study, but also for the opportunity to meet her. I told her that because of her I knew that my project was possible. Once again I saw that twinkle dancing in her eyes. I promised to come back and visit her, but she died a month later. I feel so privileged to have had the opportunity to know Lisa, even briefly. This encounter taught me a great deal about myself and has influenced my interaction with patients and the focus of my research. ∎

Judith A. DePalma, MSN, RN

LYNN

I was the supervior of the ED where Lynn was one of the staff nurses. The day before she had been brought in through our ED after a suicide attempt by drug ingestion. Our state-of-the-art medical technology had been battling to reverse Lynn's attempt to end her own life. Our technology was losing.

I went to the ED first. It was quiet; there were only four patients in the department. I then went to the ICU. The intern and resident were at Lynn's bedside. Her nurse was busy caring for her.

Lynn was in a deep coma. I could hardly recognize her through all of the equipment. I read the monitor data and knew that Lynn would not survive. Her kidneys and liver had failed from the drug overdose, so the doctors wanted to start her on dialysis. I asked if her son had been called, and was informed that he was on his way. The physicians asked me if I knew her son. I told them that I had not met him but knew that he was in his early 20s and had just become a new father 2 weeks ago.

The staff from the ED were coming up to say their good-byes to their colleague and friend. We hugged each other and comforted ourselves with warm memories of how Lynn had touched each of us.

A group of us stood together and prayed at her bedside.

I asked the doctors to be kind to Lynn and not to start her on dialysis. It was not going to change the inevitable.

Lynn's son Sean arrived. I introduced myself to him and took his hand. He had tears in his eyes. Sean was hesitant to ask questions. He was alone. His wife was at home with their newborn daughter. The intern spoke to Sean in very technical terms. The young physician struggled to find the right words so that Sean could understand. I looked at Sean and said "Your mother is going to die, Sean. There is nothing more we can offer her now to reverse the course of her actions and change the fact that she is going to die."

His tears were uncontrollable. I held him and told him how sorry I was. Tears streamed down both our faces. I told him that he needed to make decisions for his mother. He took a deep breath and asked "What needs to be done?" He would need to decide what to do if her heart stopped beating. Would he want all of the heroic measures to attempt to prolong her life or would he want us to make her comfortable and ease her passing? He looked at me and asked "What would you do?" I told him, "I would try to make the best decision for Lynn. I would make her comfortable." I was always taught that the role of the registered nurse was that of patient advocate; it was the only way I could answer.

He raised his head and said that he was sure that his mother would not want to be kept on machines. He wanted her to be comfortable. We went into the room and sat by her side. He put his head on her chest and wept.

He told me many stories of his mother. He laughed at some and cried at others. He told me of her history of depression and that she had stopped taking her medications months earlier. She was a nurse. She had worked in emergency departments all over the country. I knew her as a skilled clinician, and a compassionate, warm, funny woman who would regale the night shift with humorous anecdotes of emergency room experiences that she had during her 24-year career. She had cared for thousands of patients with self-inflicted injuries. She would recite psychiatric referrals by memory for patients in her care. She listened and directed others to seek help. She never asked for help for herself.

Lynn's heart stopped beating at 4:36 am. She passed quietly. It was peaceful in the room. I had never felt such a level of comfort with death before.

I helped to make some arrangements with Sean and a local funeral home. He hugged me and said "Thank you for being with me." I walked him to his car and watched him leave.

At the memorial service 4 days later, he turned to see me and smiled. "I didn't know if you were coming," he said. I smiled at him and offered a hug. He looked at me and said, "You will never know how much it meant to me to have you there that night. You told me the truth. The doctors didn't seem to know what to say to me. I can't thank you enough."

In my heart I knew that this was a defining moment in my nursing career. I had done the best that I could for my patient and for her son. I chose to become a registered nurse because I knew that I would be able to learn the skills necessary to become a proficient clinician. I know that I can make a difference in the lives of others because of the loss of one. ∎

Mary E. Prehoden, RN
1989

JAKE

I first heard about Jake through the nurses' expressions of sympathy about the terrible damage he had done to his esophagus and the many surgeries and extensive nursing care he would require. Soon, however, the staff began to complain in the weekly nursing care planning meetings about Jake's anger, hostility, withdrawal, and lack of appreciation.

Five months out of graduate school, I was a novice again after a decade as a nurse, creating a new psychiatric consultation liaison nursing role in a teaching hospital. I explained to the nurses that I was there to support them in stressful times and to be a resource for the psychological aspects of patient care. Jake would challenge all our routines.

Jake was a 23-year-old blond man with appealing looks. He came in after drinking Drano in a suicide attempt. He was so scared he insisted on using an alias on his medical record. As he later explained, he had been terrified that the people he believed to be chasing him would kill him. He tried to kill himself to stop his fear and anxiety.

Jake was admitted to the hospital with lye burns to his mouth, throat, esophagus, and stomach. Over the next 7 months, he underwent approximately 15 surgical proce-

dures including a tracheostomy, a gastrostomy, and creating a new esophagus from his stomach. He needed extensive nursing care for problems such as nausea and vomiting, coughing, excessive secretions, inadequate nutrition, and difficulty tolerating foods by mouth. In addition, he demonstrated anger, anxiety, fear, and depression, and he struggled with the staff about his participation in his care.

I listened to the staff. "Here is this guy who did it to himself. Why should we spend so much time caring for someone who doesn't like us, is nasty, hostile, unappreciative, and coughs sputum everywhere?" Despite their feelings, the staff made a connection with Jake. I met with them weekly, supporting their connection with him, acknowledging their feelings, planning care that demonstrated caring concern, limit-setting, and helping them face such extreme breakdown. Together, we created a caring community around Jake.

Jake could only communicate in writing because of the tracheostomy. If he chose to write, he wrote on a magic pad that he could erase easily. If he didn't want to communicate, he would close his eyes and simply refuse. He ignored me. I said "I'm here if you want to talk. I'll be here for ____ minutes. When I leave, I will be back tomorrow." He let me know that he did not want anything to do with anyone associated with psychiatry.

Throughout the many months, Jake controlled the direction and depth of our conversation. Jake would accept nothing less than basic trust and friendship—my connection with him as a human being. Any time I ventured into 'therapeutic communication,' or tried any techniques, it came to a standstill.

Was I violating the rules of therapeutic relationships? I wasn't sure. The relationship was reduced to basic human terms. Jake was one of society's marginal people, lacking a past of enough care, attention, and responsiveness to be fully a self. I felt the stigma of association with someone disenfranchised and suffering. With patience and caring, I accepted whatever he gave—his anger, his silence, his tidbits of personal history and, later, his determination to be well. Along with the nursing staff, I remained firm about the limits. He began to trust enough to develop a relationship.

After 7 months in the hospital, Jake was discharged. He began writing letters telling all of us how he was relearning to eat, blenderizing his food, lifting weights, and getting stronger. He identified 17 nursing staff individually by name in a letter of thanks and appreciation 4 years later. He shared his excitement about being alive. In the letters, Jake revealed thoughts he'd kept to himself in the hospital. He told us of how, when he was admitted, how shocked and angry he was to wake up and find himself alive. How he made me his friend because he needed one so badly. How betrayed he felt about getting kicked out of the hospital before he felt ready. He repeated his appreciation and thanks to the "beautiful crew that kept me alive."

Reading his letters, I realized I felt like his parent—as if over the long 7 months, we gave psychological birth to his new self. That self was beginning a journey into a new life.

Ten years later, Jake returned to the hospital to create a 'Thank-You' ceremony for the staff. He gave a speech and plaques to the nurses, to the physicians, and to me. He called me "his friend for life." On the plaque he gave me, which hangs in my office, he thanked me for "being my friend when I needed one as bad as I needed you." He also thanked me "for being there, day in and day out, and for being with me though [sic] the most horrific time of my entire life." At the end of his speech to his assembled past caregivers, Jake said "You've all touched my life very deeply and through my little ceremony and the plaques, I hope to touch yours." He did. ∎

Pamela Minarik, MS, RN, CS, FAAN
1980

ANGELA

When I met 4-year-old Angela, it was to tell her why she was feeling so tired and getting bruises on her body. Angela's physician had already told her mother the diagnosis: leukemia, discovered the week after Christmas. Using terms like good cells, bad cells, and germs, I explained leukemia, bone marrow biopsy, and chemotherapy at a level I hoped Angela would understand. I tried to focus only on Angela and not on the tears quietly streaming down her mother's face.

When I asked Angela if she understood what I had told her, she looked up at me and said bravely, "I am sick and I cannot be around germs. Some things that the doctors and nurses will do to make me healthy might hurt, but you know what—I am going to get better so I can go home and open my presents from Santa." I knew then that our special bond had begun.

This became the first of many "But you know what—" conversations between us, and they became her way of sharing both the bad and the good of her illness and treatment. Angela was often bothered by nightmares and would tell me about them. However, she would follow this by saying, "But you know what—I think about angels when I have bad dreams and the dreams go away." One of the most distressing side effects of chemotherapy for Angela was the possibility that her hair could fall out. She would cover her ears and shake her head vigorously 'no' if any of the nurses mentioned this to her. In one of her proudest moments she told me, "My hair is getting thinner, but you know what—my bangs were getting so long that my mommy had to cut them."

On rare occasions, Angela's mother needed to leave the hospital for a short time, and Angela was sad. However, Angela explained to me, "My mommy had to do some errands today, but you know what—I know she is coming back because she left me her lipstick."

Many children have touched my heart, but perhaps none quite so deeply as Angela. She is a delightful and social child who warms the hearts of all of us who care for her. She shows concern for everyone and makes each of us feel as though we are her best friends, a role we truly know belongs only to her mother. That does not stop her from sometimes climbing up on my lap, giving me a hug, and whispering in my ear, "But you know what, I love you." You know what Angela, I love you too. ∎

Michele Prior, MSN, RN
1997

REGGIE

I was working the night shift as a traveling nurse on a 16-bed AIDS care unit. Reggie was admitted from ED just before the change of shifts. I was assigned to care for him and also the three other men in his room. In report, the day nurse told me that he was a 24-year-old male just admitted from ED with possible pneumocystis pneumonia (PCP). He had been in ED since early that morning with high fevers and shortness of breath. The resident said his chest x-ray looked 'weird' and was highly suspicious for PCP. The patient reported a history of 10-pound weight loss, anorexia, diarrhea, fever, and general malaise for the past 2 weeks—all of these, symptoms of PCP. His temperature was now 102°F, and oxygen saturation level was 94% on room air. His risk factor was unknown. He had never been HIV tested.

When I first saw Reggie, he was sitting up in bed eating a sandwich and chips. He was laughing and talking with the other three patients in the room and in no apparent distress. He was a handsome Hispanic man, who looked much younger than his 24 years. I introduced myself, did a quick assessment, and told him I'd be back later to give him his medications.

I returned to his room and then left the room briefly to mix his IV

Septra. When I returned, Reggie was in tears. When I asked why he was upset, he wouldn't answer. I went about my business, telling him that I would be on all night and that I would be checking in on him from time to time. The next time I made rounds, the other three patients were asleep. Reggie was wide awake and watching TV. When I asked how he was feeling, the tears started to flow. "I'm so scared!" he cried. "The doctors all think I have PCP; if I do, that means that I have AIDS! They took blood in the ED to test me for HIV!"

In the course of the next few minutes he told me that he was from a large Hispanic family who would surely disown him if it turned out that he had AIDS. He had been working as an auto mechanic in the family business. He had successfully hidden the fact that he was gay from his entire family. He was sure that they would no longer have anything to do with him if they found out his sexual orientation. I tried my best to console him, to no avail. It was a long, frustrating night for me. By morning, Reggie had convinced himself that he had the flu, was now better, and that everything would be just fine.

I didn't see Reggie again until 4 months later when he was admitted to our ward with wasting syndrome. He was painfully thin. He still had not told his family of his diagnosis. They were becoming suspicious, and he was going to have to tell them sometime very soon. He said that he was so afraid that they would never see or speak to him again. Again, I tried to reassure him that sometimes people are surprising and things may not turn out as badly as he might think.

In the course of the next few months, Reggie was a patient on our ward many times for many different HIV-related illnesses. He became a favorite of all the nurses on the ward. He was one of our youngest patients, and we all called him 'our baby.' With each admission, the nurses watched his health decline. He had finally summoned the courage to tell his family and, true to his expectations, they abandoned him. His only visitors were a few close friends.

One Thursday night, I was receiving report when the day shift nurse told me "Reggie is really going downhill fast—he doesn't seem to have any fight left in him." We gave each other that knowing look that meant that the end was near. I selfishly hoped that he wouldn't go on my shift—I wasn't sure I could emotionally take his death. All the nurses had known Reggie since that first admission and had worked with him through his physical decline, as well as the emotional upheaval with his family. We knew he was alone in the world.

The shift was uneventful until about 3 am, when I was making rounds. I found Reggie awake and grimacing in pain. He had severe Kaposi's sarcoma (KS) lesions on both of his lower legs. The KS, coupled with severe neuropathy, was causing him intense pain. He asked me if he could have a 'shot for the pain.' I called the night-float intern, who ordered morphine 4 mg IM. I took the injection back into the room. When I told Reggie that it was an injection, he started to cry. "I can't stand any more pain—can't you put it in the IV?"

After much convincing and pleading, the intern agreed to let me IV push the morphine. Reggie grabbed my hand and asked me if we could talk for awhile. He asked me if I was working over the weekend. I told him that I would be off. He asked if I had any big plans. We talked briefly about my plans, then he said "You know I think I'm probably going to have a good weekend too; I'm pretty sure that I'm going to die this weekend. I just wanted to thank you for always being so nice to me." I looked down at this sweet, brave, young man and fought back tears. I said "Reggie, I'll never forget you—you've been nice to me too." I left the room, went out to the desk, put my head down, and wept.

When I went to work on Monday night, I peeked into the room that Reggie had been in. Someone else was in that bed. I asked the day nurse when Reggie had died. She told me he had died the previous night on the night shift. 'Our baby' had died alone with only his nurse at his bedside. ∎

Jill Kunkel, RN
1991

FARIDA

Pinocchio was Farida's favorite children's video. I set it up so Farida and her 16-year-old sister, Salwa, could watch the story while I was nearby answering telephones, charting, figuring out staffing, and planning a care conference. I was caught off guard when I felt 5-year-old Farida's arms around me, her head on my chest and the softly spoken words, "You're my best friend." These were the first English words she had ever spoken to me. Her family was Middle Eastern and had been in the U.S. for only 4 years before they had to rush this very ill, little, curly-haired, big-brown-eyed child to the hospital. She was diagnosed with new onset diabetes.

Initially Farida was in and out of consciousness. Her father and 14-year-old sister Soad stood by her side, scared and silent. Within 24 hours Farida was awake, alert, she began to eat, and her insulin drip was discontinued. Now came the most challenging teaching dilemma of my 20-year career. This loving family needed to understand that Farida had a life-long disease that would require them to precisely measure her food, activity levels, blood sugar levels, give her insulin injections, and balance all this around the clock.

Our care conference involved a compassionate team of nurses, doctors, social workers, home health nurses, diabetic educators, dieticians, and Arabic interpreters. We had come to an understanding about this family that was weighing heavily on our hearts and minds. Dad was the only family member with a full education. School-age siblings had been in school for 2 years already and Mom had never been to school. Shortly after the family teachings had begun, Mom removed herself and stated, "I am her mother. I cannot do this." Her daily visits of an hour or two were those of a mother's love and tenderness. Dad was catching on to our teachings like a scholar, but his employment often took him from the home.

Who could Farida rely on to check her blood sugar at dinnertime and give her life-sustaining insulin injections? Salwa and Soad, her sisters and guardian angels, were to be the focus of our teachings! Willing, receptive to our teachings, and devoted to their little sister, both learned how to prick Farida's little fingers and perform the Accuchecks to test her blood sugar.

Now was the horrendous task of teaching them how to draw up and give insulin. They had watched the videos and seen the nurses. They had witnessed Farida's rage following the injections. Salwa and Soad took turns staying with, playing with, and sleeping beside Farida. I chose Salwa, the eldest sister, first. She thought she was ready. Salwa precisely drew up the regular insulin and then the NPH. She prepped Farida's skinny thigh with alcohol. Salwa took one last look into Farida's big brown eyes and then liquefied. With her head down, she handed me the syringe and softly stated, "I'm sorry, I cannot." I tried to reassure Salwa that it was OK and I quickly gave the injection. True to form, Farida stormed the hallways, feet stomping, arms flailing, tears rolling, with screams of protest.

Like her older sister, Soad skillfully performed the Accucheck and prepared the insulin syringe. I held Farida snuggly and Soad asked "Did my sister Salwa do this?" I said, "No, and if you can't, that's OK, but I think you can." My fearful thought was "What will we do if she can't?"

With bold tenderness she did it! Soad did it! Our sad yet courageous moment of triumph was here! Farida's disbelieving silence lasted maybe 5 seconds before her rage followed. This time toys flew, trash cans were flipped, and chairs turned over. She tore at Soad's clothes, pulling off Soad's scarf (I was delighted to finally see the full head of soft curls that framed this beautiful young woman's face) as her screams escalated. Soad and I were both frozen in disbelief and yet silently celebrating our victory. It was this 14-year-old's bold love and understanding that led her to the next natural reaction. Soad scooped up Farida into her arms and embarrassed her with a tenderness that I will never forget and felt honored to witness.

The next day at the changing of the guard, Soad beamed with pride as she shared the events with her big sister and father. Salwa was quick to follow her little sister's lead and we were able to soon discharge this family.

During those days, thoughts of little Farida, courageous Salwa, and tender Soad stayed with me. What became of Farida's rage I'll never know. I do know that like Pinocchio, she had been to a scary place and found her way back home to her loving and supportive family. I know I can make a wish that she have a really happy and healthy childhood and I believe it will come true. ∎

Kathy Springer, RN
1998

DONNA

The importance of holistic nursing is so apparent to me. Our mental well-being and physical well-being are intertwined.

I was assured Donna would be one of my easiest patients. Yet, while assessing Donna, I noticed she would not make direct eye contact. During my shift, she called out every 3 to 4 hours for pain injections. She kept her back turned away from the door. At times, I thought I heard muffled sounds of crying.

Once, while passing her room, I heard her arguing and crying with someone on the phone. After her conversation ended, I spoke with her. I told her that I felt something other than pain was bothering her. She told me she was worried about her 12-year-old daughter, who was staying with her mother while she was in the hospital.

Donna asked me what shifts I worked and whether I had any children. As we spoke, she seemed to relax and become less tearful. I sat down and took her hand, looked into her eyes, and asked her once again what was really bothering her. She then told me her story.

It was a story of how her husband physically abused her and threatened that he would take her daughter. She was afraid that while she was in the hospital he would carry out his threat. I reassured her and allowed her to talk. I suggested several agencies that would assist her.

I shared with her that she was not alone. At this time we both had tears in our eyes and her trust in me was apparent. We both shared an inner peace. She no longer cried or laid with her back to the door. Requests for pain medication ceased. Throughout the rest of my 16 hours, we continued to talk and joke until she was able to smile.

When I returned to work a week later, she had left a 3x5 painting of a faceless nurse holding a heart in one hand and a flower in the other. There was an inscription stating "Nursing is the gentle art of caring," along with a thank-you card saying:

`Dear Rachel,

Thank you again for being that one-in-a-million person and going out of your way to care when others need it—both physically and emotionally. People like you only come once in a lifetime. I thank God you were in mine.'

This was probably the greatest gift I could have received: recognition of who I am and what I do as both a person and a nurse. ■

Rachel Briston-Griffin, BSN, RN
1992

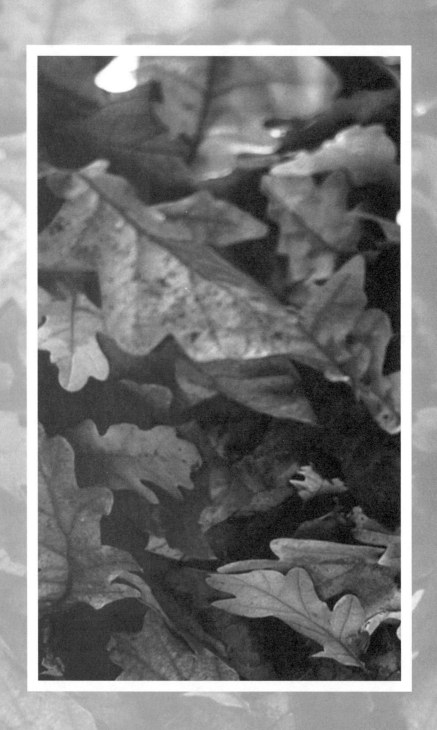

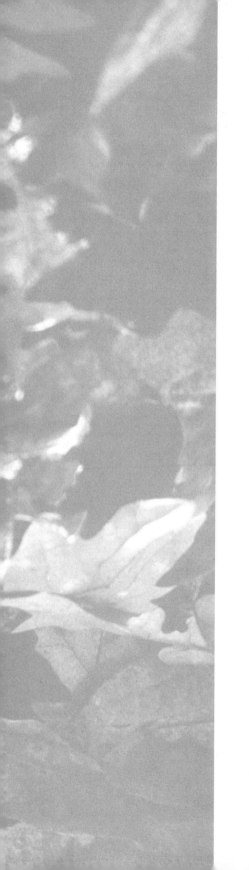

FAITH

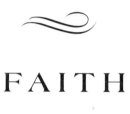

BETH

Saturday morning on the general surgery/trauma unit. You never know what to expect on weekends, especially in the summer. I had been assigned an 18-year-old named Beth. A drunk driver had run Beth off the road the night before. She had been working the late shift at a local restaurant and was on her way home. She was scheduled to go to the OR during my shift to have her broken jaw repaired. She was lucky that was the only thing broken, but she had sustained many bruises.

I entered Beth's room to prepare her for surgery. Beth's face was very swollen and her eyes were just slits. Most of her face was now multicolored—purple, black, and red from the bruises. The night nurses had taped a plastic sheet over her mirror to give her time to get over the trauma. I introduced myself and told her I would be her primary nurse. Beth was quiet. Her family came in: mom, dad, and two younger siblings. Mom had brought Beth's prom pictures in from the week before. Beth looked beautiful in the pictures. Although Beth's injuries were not high on the life-threatening scale, I couldn't help but feel empathy for someone at her age to have to go through this. The end of senior year is supposed to be a milestone in one's life and a time

for celebration. I could also tell that her parents were trying to control their anger at a driver who was so careless.

Beth went through surgery without any problems. The surgeons wired her jaw shut to allow the fractures to heal and repaired the deep scars on her face. I got to know Beth and her family a little more each day as I worked with them. Eventually we took the cover off the mirror. We emphasized to Beth that her face would return to its usual state once the swelling went down. She handled it quite stoically. Beth's graduation was the following Saturday and she told us she wanted to go. Her parents looked to the surgeons and me for advice. Beth wasn't eating yet and she was still a little unsteady on her feet. Yet both the surgeons and I knew it was important for her to go, and we agreed to let her out on a pass for a few hours to attend her graduation.

Beth and her parents were excited. I could tell, however, that her parents were also nervous taking their daughter out of the hospital so soon. I discussed with my nurse manager, Nancy, that I wanted to go with Beth to her graduation to make sure she would be okay and ease the stress for her parents. Nancy understood my wanting to go, but voiced her concern that I did not have my own malpractice insurance to cover me once I left the hospital. Nursing leadership reviewed the case, and they agreed to give me extended coverage so I could go to the graduation.

It was all set. The day of graduation I helped Beth dress in her cap and gown. It was one of those hot and humid days, 95° outside, and it felt like walking through a soggy sponge. I packed emergency IV fluids and brought a pair of wire cutters in case Beth became nauseous and I had to release her jaw.

Beth's hardworking father spared no expense for his daughter and rented a stretch limousine for the day. As I wheeled Beth out of the hospital in her cap and gown, the staff applauded. Some attempted to sing the graduation theme song. The graduation ceremony was held outside, so we waited in the air-conditioned limousine until it was just about ready to begin. Once the music started, I wheeled Beth to her seat and I sat next to her. When her name was called, she insisted on walking up to the podium; I just held her arm and tried to be invisible. She received a standing ovation from her classmates. The goodwill in the crowd was palpable, and I was not the only one in the crowd who was a little teary. Beth had demonstrated such resilience.

As we drove back to the hospital, Beth and her family were ecstatic that the day turned out so well. The importance of social support as it relates to wellness is well documented in the health literature. I didn't need a study to tell me how important it was on that graduation day. ■

Susan Allison, MS, RN, CS, CETN
1989

MILAGRO

It was 11:00 pm, Christmas Eve. I was a student nurse and my role on OB was to scrub in, be available to the obstetrician, and do as I was told. As I entered the unit, I felt a heavy blanket of silence everywhere. No one was smiling and the doctor seemed indescribably nervous. "Mrs. Nielsen is in labor and due to deliver at any moment...I wish I were off duty...I dread this evening" were some of the statements I heard from the nurses as I entered the room for report.

Marianne Nielsen was a 45-year-old woman, pregnant for the 18th time, but with no living children. The doctors had advised Mrs. Nielsen that for her own health and well-being, she should consider having her tubes tied following this pregnancy. The Nielsens wanted a child so very much, and Marianne had been pregnant every other year since their marriage. Each of her past 17 pregnancies had ended in an early, spontaneous abortion or the infant had died at some time prior to delivery. Modern medicine had tried everything within its power, but had been unable to save any infant or prevent the miscarriages.

As we were concluding report, one of the labor room nurses reported that Mrs. Nielsen was ready to deliver. "Warner, hop to it, scrub and get into Room 2 immediately." "Oh no" I thought. "What do I do—I can't bear to be in that room if this mother loses another child!" I stood at the end of the table and watched as Mrs. Nielsen was being rolled into the labor room. I prayed silently, "Oh dear God, spare this child, may we witness a miracle." As though I had been heard, Mrs. Nielsen looked at me and smiled. "Birth is truly a miracle from God you know." I blinked hard and swallowed, hoping to diminish the lump in my throat. "Yes, Mrs. Nielsen, miracles are from God and I believe in miracles." It was difficult to speak through my mask, but she understood as she locked eyes with me and answered, "Yes, so do I," as though we formed a secret pact.

The medical team defended itself with the activities of prepping, draping, IVs, sterile fields and used these effectively as shields to avoid any conversation. Mrs. Nielsen knew quite well what to do by now. She needed little instruction. As the baby's head began to crown, the doctor took a deep breath and said "Please, dear God." All I could do was pray as never before. One more push and the baby's head emerged. The doctor immediately suctioned the baby's air passage and felt around the neck for a possible entwined umbilical cord. He looked at me and his eyes said what we were all thinking—"so far so good."

With another contraction, the body slipped out into the doctor's arms. He moved quickly, holding the baby by its ankles and stimulating that long-anticipated cry. Those few seconds passed like hours. Everyone's eyes focused on the baby. We all held our breath awaiting the infant's first breath. Perspiration formed on the doctor's brow as he said "Breathe, little one."

Just as the doctor was about to begin more aggressive measures, there was a loud cry, followed by cheers and tears from the multitudes then gathered in the delivery room. "It's a girl—a beautiful, healthy, living baby girl," the doctor's voice was almost melodious.

"Thank you, oh thank you, God" was all I could think. The sobs of joy consumed the room as Mrs. Nielsen held her baby, stroking the child gently, and smiling as tears streamed down her cheeks.

I could barely see through my own tears. "Mrs. Nielsen, do you have a name picked out for your daughter?" I asked. "Oh yes, her name will be called Milagro, for indeed she is a miracle."

I always remember how on that Christmas Eve of 1961, I participated in hope, faith, and in what some might call a "milagro." ∎

Carmen Germaine Warner,
MSN, RN, FAAN
1961

SEAN

Everyone who is a nurse expects calls from neighbors about health care. Sometimes there is an emergency. Every nurse feels some responsibility for the health of her community and is willing to help where possible, despite cautions we have received about "practicing beyond the scope of our practice." One day I received such a call.

I had just come home from returning a video, when my husband told me a toddler was missing. I joined the other neighbors in looking for the lost 2-year-old boy. We found him quickly—face down, blue and lifeless in a neighbor's pool. I jumped in the pool and waded out to him. As I lifted his unmoving body into my arms, my 11 years of nursing experience in intensive care told me this child was dead. However, I was a CPR instructor and I automatically began cardiopulmonary resuscitation.

For almost 30 minutes I continued breathing and compressions. There was no response. The ambulance came, but a voice in my head told me "keep doing CPR, don't stop." I looked down and saw that I had been giving adult lung volumes, and air had escaped from the child's lungs into his stomach, making it distended. I compressed the stomach, using the Heimlich maneuver, and the little boy regurgitated. At that moment, his pulse returned! He was, however, still not breathing. I held him in my arms and continued rescue breathing, refusing to let the teenaged ambulance attendant take him.

I climbed in my neighbor's car, the owner of the pool. As she drove 100 miles per hour to the hospital, I continued mouth-to-mouth breathing. The little boy's color was improving. As we pulled into the ER parking lot, he took a little breath, almost like a sigh. I ran into the trauma room and pulled 100% oxygen off the wall, screaming to the physician to start an IV and get a blood gas.

I don't want to tell you what I said when they told me to go to the desk to fill out the paperwork. I didn't leave. The first blood gas confirmed my suspicion that the child had been clinically dead. His color rapidly improved, and after 30 minutes, his eyes opened, and in a hoarse voice he said "potty."

I'm grateful I am a nurse and was able to serve. I'm glad I didn't care about 'scope of practice' or being 'just a nurse' and that I listened to that voice. I am glad to say that little boy is fine today. He's 11 years old and gifted in math. He seems to have an unnatural sensitivity and perceptiveness to the needs of others. I've kept close tabs on him during the years, for, you see, he is my only child, my son Sean. ∎

Maria Lasater, MSN, RN, CCRN
1989

HARRY AND CLAIRE

I had been working as a registered nurse for a little over a year in the intermediate step-down unit. I suctioned Harry and decided to bathe him because it was already 4 am, and I thought I'd have him 'fluffed and buffed' by the change of shift.

Harry and I spent many Saturday nights together. We had CNN on and the lights dimmed while I chattered to this 69-year-old man who was far away from home. He and his wife Claire had been driving through Pittsburgh in their Winnebago, fulfilling a dream to travel throughout the United States.

On a cool March morning, Harry and Claire stopped to 'gas up' the Winnebago and have breakfast before moving on to Washington, DC to see the cherry blossoms in bloom. As the two began to drive out of the gas station, Harry clutched his chest and, putting the Winnebago in park, lost consciousness.

Alone in a strange city without family or friends, Claire called 911, described their situation, and waited for help. The paramedics arrived, stabilized Harry, and took both of them to the hospital. After an unsuccessful angioplasty of his coronary blood vessels, Harry was sent to the OR for emergency coronary bypass surgery. Harry never regained consciousness. He was put on a ventilator. The calendar changed. Harry's chest wounds had healed, and Claire continued to sit faithfully by his side day after day, but Harry was still asleep 61 days later.

I bathed Harry as I continued my one-sided conversation with him about my diabetic dog. I washed his arm and washed carefully in between each and every finger, and then I respectfully asked Harry to hold his arm up so that I could wash under it, though I knew he couldn't hear me. This evening was different for Harry and me though. This time when I asked him to hold up his arm, I could feel his arm straighten and stiffen. I let go of his wrist and his arm stayed in the air! With tears in my eyes, I asked Harry if he could hear me, but his eyes remained shut and his facial expression was unchanged. I then asked him to squeeze my hand and he did.

By the end of the week Harry was awake and following commands. Eleven weeks after surgery, Harry's tracheostomy tube had been capped and he began to whisper. Harry asked where he was, and where was Claire, his wife and best friend for 37 years. We had been chatting for an hour when he looked at me with his deep blue eyes and asked me how my dog was. Stories about my diabetic dog, Marti's little girl, Dr. Rich's fishing trip, and details about a surprise spring snow began pouring from his lips. I've had patients tell me stories that they had remembered hearing while asleep, but never did a patient remember so many different stories in so much detail. After 77 days, Harry and Claire walked out of the hospital together to go home to Oregon to recuperate.

Nine years have passed since I met Harry, and I continue to talk to my patients about the weather, world issues, their family, and what has been happening on my favorite television shows, even though my patients may be unconscious or unable to clearly understand the words.

I know that my patients can hear me speak hopeful words. They can feel me touch them with caring hands, and they know, for that moment, that I am caring only about them while I wait for them to wake from a sleep that cannot always end. ∎

Karen A. Tarolli, BSN, RN
1989

HELEN

On the evening shift in the NICU, my patient was Helen, a term infant born to a first-time mother. She had spent her first 8 hours with her mom, feeding and acting like a normal newborn. After 8 hours, she was brought to the NICU for worsening episodes of apnea and dusky discoloration of the skin. She was placed on mechanical ventilation after an increase in number and intensity of these episodes.

Helen began to have seizures despite anticonvulsant medications. She was in *status epilepticus*. The only way the seizures could be stopped was with the paralyzing agent curare. Helen had a very grim prognosis. A CAT scan revealed a right cerebral artery infarct consistent with a diagnosis of a prenatal stroke. The parents were devastated. The mother was an RN, and clearly understood the implications of the diagnosis. In an effort to protect the mom, the father was struggling with the difficult decision of discontinuing the mechanical ventilation to see if Helen could breathe on her own. The curare was discontinued so she could try to resume her own respirations.

Renee C. Grieger, BSN, RN
1981

The father was desperate for an answer, which no one could give him. We spent a long time together...we sat quietly. We talked, we cried, we prayed, and when the time was right we took Helen off the ventilator. She began to breathe on her own and improved slowly, with increased alertness and responsiveness. Within the next few days she began to feed, displaying a good suck-swallow reflex.

On day 16 of life Helen was discharged from the hospital on medication. She had a definite left hemiparesis for which she would be followed. It wouldn't be an easy course for Helen, but I knew that her parents would develop her to her greatest potential. I lost contact with Helen. Years later, she appeared in the NICU with her Mom. She hugged me and announced that she had won the 4th grade mathematics award in 'regular' school. We took a picture of her, which I keep in my daily planner as a reminder of this miracle.

I am grateful to all the patients and their families of the past 20 years. They have given me so much, yet they come to thank me. As nurses we have the unique opportunity to witness miracles, and Helen certainly is one that I find myself drawing on frequently for strength and insight.

'Hopeless' is not a word that should be spoken in the NICU, and I do not accept it easily. Helen was the restoration of faith in those things that are out of our control. ∎

GREGG

This was my 8th year of teaching undergraduate psychiatric–mental health nursing clinical practicums on the inpatient units. I always seemed to get at least one or two students who 'hate' psych or had judgments toward patients diagnosed with drug or alcohol abuse. This semester brought one of my biggest challenges, in a student named Gregg. He was extremely bright, conscientious, and self-disciplined. He had trained for a triathlon and, by a quirk of fate, was assigned to the chemical dependency unit. His assignment was to choose a patient for group and one-to-one interactions and then to write up a plan of care.

It didn't take long for me to learn that this was a poor match. Gregg just couldn't grasp why these patients were using drugs or alcohol. "Don't they see how harmful it is?" he would ask me. He couldn't see the point of empathic 'listening' and allowing people to vent their feelings. He believed that what he should do is "just tell them what to do and how to straighten out their lives." Gregg knew he had the answers and just wanted patients to do as he told them. He also couldn't understand the 12-step program. To Gregg, it was all a lack of willpower.

So, every week I sat down with Gregg. I tried to explain different theories of drug and alcohol treatment. More importantly, I hoped he could realize the importance of 'active listening' and developing a therapeutic approach with patients. I explained that this would apply everywhere in nursing, to every patient and to every person he would encounter in his life, not just on this psych unit. Each time, he countered my explanations with arguments. Each week we had lively discussions and provocative dialogues about our different perspectives. By the end of the semester, he completed the course with a passing grade, but I was not convinced that he understood my teaching and the very healing value of *listening*.

The semester ended. Gregg went on to his next year's classes. I periodically saw him in the hallways of the nursing school. One day, he came up to me excitedly. "Professor Bormann, you were right! I kept thinking of what you were saying about the importance of listening to patients before telling them what to do. So I decided to try it. It works! I had this patient in the ICU and he just needed to talk. So I kept my mouth shut and just listened. He thanked me over and over again, just for listening and being there for him. I just had to tell you. Thanks again for being so patient with me on the psych unit." I felt a tingle down my spine. ∎

Jill Bormann, PhD, RN, CS
1989

SYLVANA

Early one morning, as I was performing rounds as a nurse midwife with residents at a large women's hospital, I met Sylvana. She seemed so tiny, just lying in bed on the labor and delivery unit. She had intravenous lines in, various pumps with medications, and she was attached to an external fetal monitor. What I had learned from her history was that she had had a prior Cesarean section in Central America and during the time just prior to the C-section or immediately following, her infant had died. She spoke only Spanish.

I introduced myself to her on rounds and asked if she was in pain. She only 'held me with her eyes' and nodded that she was fine. I asked her if she would like to consider any pain medication or an epidural analgesia. Again, she indicated "no" and spoke in Spanish, saying she did not want anything placed into her back.

Throughout the morning, she made very slow progress in terms of dilatation of the cervix and descent of the fetus. She couldn't tell me much about the loss of her previous child as she did not know many of the details. I said to her "This must be an important pregnancy and baby for you now." She looked up at me and smiled and nodded "yes." Her eyes filled up, yet she still said nothing.

Hours went by and I would enter her room to read the fetal monitor or examine her cervix. Sylvana seemed adamant about not taking any medication. I finally convinced her that she seemed to have many more hours of labor and could benefit from taking some pain medication for relief. She nodded in agreement. The intravenous medication helped her sleep between contractions. I was in and out of her room, examining the fetal tracing and applying scalp stimulation to the fetus for reassurance that there was no fetal distress. During all of these exams and extensive monitoring, Sylvana would always nod her approval. When we explained why we were doing things, she would nod "yes" that she understood. An interpreter also explained events to her, and she seemed to accept everything passively.

Her infant was posterior and caused her increased backache and discomfort. When asked again if she wanted pain medication or anesthesia, she indicated "no." The father of this baby finally came to visit her. He quietly sat in his chair next to her. They said very little to each other. I spoke with him through an interpreter, and he explained that they were both nervous about the outcome since she had had 'problems' with the last baby. He didn't know any specifics about the death of that infant, either.

Slowly, Sylvana began to make progress to full dilatation and began to push. This went on for 3 hours. Although this baby was not very big, it had to rotate from being posterior.

I've never seen anyone try so hard to push and to accommodate to anything you asked of her as Sylvana. I told her how critical it was to maximize each pushing effort since the infant needed to descend more, and she also had to rotate the baby's head as well. She had never delivered an infant vaginally, and I could tell how critical it was for her to participate in her birth, deliver this baby vaginally, and produce a good outcome. She and I worked hard as a team through each contraction. My presence and persistent support and encouragement helped her to keep going.

I pushed with her for 3 hours. Sylvana was beginning to become exhausted. I assisted her with different positions for pushing, examining the infant's monitor tracing and performing cervical exams. Her efforts finally began to bring the infant down the birth canal and rotate. By now, 10½ hours had gone by. It was my time to leave for the day. I had to explain to her in Spanish that even though I had been there all this time, someone else would be taking over for me. As I told her in Spanish, her eyes got wide and she stiffened in the bed. Yet she said nothing. She reached out for my hand, grabbed it and said "Thank you." These were her only words the entire day. They said so much. She had trusted me to help her through this and although she found it hard for me to leave, she was very grateful.

An hour later, she went on to deliver a male infant by forceps. It was a slightly difficult delivery. Her baby was sent to neonatal ICU for observation, and did well. ∎

Diane J. Angelini, EdD, RN, CNM, CNAA, FACNM
1998

JASON

When I first saw Jason, he was lying flat on his back in the neurological ward of the hospital where I was a psychiatric clinical nurse specialist. He was paralyzed and unable to speak, sliding in and out of consciousness. The diagnosis was Guillian-Barré syndrome, which he had contracted months before, following a bacterial infection with a high fever. He had just been weaned from the respirator that had been breathing for him for the past 3 months and had been transferred to a step down unit. His prognosis was poor; the disease had taken a heavy toll. He had no family or friends. No one came to visit or be his advocate for care.

I was often called to see patients and staff who were having a particularly stressful time in the hospital. In addition to listening, I also did a number of touch therapies to calm and reduce tension. In my work, I found acupressure to be particularly helpful easing pain, reducing muscle spasms, and aiding neurological functioning. When I overheard one of the nurses in report saying that Jason was "the same as usual—no change," I decided to pay him a visit, thinking that perhaps the acupressure and my contact could help make a difference.

I don't know what I expected to do for him, maybe make some magic, create some dramatic change. So I went in and introduced myself and explained about acupressure and what I wanted to do even though he was unresponsive. Thus began a daily visit to his bedside, with me coming in and doing acupressure on him for about half an hour. During this time, Jason remained nonverbal and unresponsive. As time went on, I found myself becoming increasing downhearted, doubting that anything was really happening during my visits. However, I did not stop. There was no one else visiting and occasionally he seemed to recognize me. I believed someone regularly giving him attention could be healing and could let the staff see that he was not completely forgotten.

As the months went by and he remained essentially the same, it became increasingly harder to visit him. I wondered what I was really doing for him, having given up hope that the acupressure would create any form of change.

One day I came to the unit to find he had been transferred to a chronic long-term unit. With a sense of growing despair, I went to the unit and introduced myself to the head nurse, telling her about my visits and my interest in his care. I hoped she too would share in my involvement. She seemed like a no-nonsense kind of person who, while strict, was conscientious and dedicated to her patients. I continued to visit but not as often as before because the head nurse began an active physical program with him, combining range-of-motion exercises with continuous encouragement and verbal stimulation. Under her nursing care, I watched him slowly respond and felt happy on the one hand to see his improvement while a little jealous that it was not me who had created the change.

In the months that followed, I saw Jason slowly return to awareness and to activity. He began to speak, sit up, and eventually learn to walk again. He seemed to need the activity that the unit provided and his relationship with the head nurse seemed very warm and supportive. I felt in a way I had held his hand until she was able to get in there and work with him actively.

Whenever I came on the unit, he welcomed me warmly, anxious to show me the new things he was able to do. We spent more time talking now—about his life and his future and what he wanted to do once he left the hospital. Sometimes we'd talk about the past and what life was like prior to his illness. One day we began to talk about his time on the step down unit, and I realized how aware he was even though he was unable to communicate at that time. I said "I used to come and visit and do my acupressure, but I never really knew if you even knew I was there." He said "I used to lie there listening to my breathing, scared that at any moment it might stop. Then you'd come in and you'd work on me and I could breathe more easily. It helped me survive another day." Listening to Jason I realized that you don't always know what impact you might have. Frequently your impact is very different from what you've intended. Jason helped me let go of the outcome and just enjoy the process, trusting that we would get to where we needed to be—through faith. ∎

Mary Anne LaTorre, MA, RN, CNS
1981

LI HUA

The setting was the largest psychiatric hospital in China. In 1988 I left Seattle to determine if I would marry the man who is now my husband, a Canadian psychiatrist/anthropologist committed to teaching and research work in China. My 6-month trial period has led to more than 10 years in China. We had moved to a 1,500-bed hospital in Beijing.

So on this morning I was not taken aback to see patients dressed in blue-and-white uniforms, living on locked wards, and being herded about in groups. My intent was to observe a head nurse conduct a patient interview with the skills she had learned in my communications class.

The patient chosen for the interview, Li Hua, was disheveled and expressionless as she entered the room. I was intrigued because she was clutching a Bible to her chest, a sight rarely seen in China. The head nurse told me since Li Hua's hospitalization 1 week earlier, she had been extremely anxious, had neither eaten nor spoken much, and was easily startled by men, including her male doctor. This was her first psychiatric hospitalization. She had been diagnosed with schizophrenia. For several months, she had believed that someone wanted to kill her, had heard voices

of someone telling her she would die, and often had repetitive nightmares in which she woke up shouting.

Li Hua's hands trembled and her legs jerked. Her speech was slow and slurred. She asked for a cigarette and then later, to hold my hand. "Can I talk to you in English?" was her next question. I was quite curious, so with the head nurse's consent, I took over the interview. I asked "Where did you learn English?" "Argentina" she said, to my surprise. With a few prompting questions, she told her story in a mix of English and Chinese.

Li Hua came from a wealthy Beijing family of five. Because of her epilepsy, she and her family realized she would not easily find a husband. So at 28, rather than marrying the man of her choice, she consented to marry a man chosen by her father. He was her father's employee and 12 years her senior.

Shortly after their marriage she discovered her husband had a girlfriend. While Li Hua was hospitalized for tuberculosis, he took all of her money and went to Argentina. One year later, when the money was spent, he called and asked her to come to Argentina. She resisted, but her mother insisted, "You married him, you must go."

She went to Argentina. Friends had warned her of her husband's plan to sell her, but she would not believe it until, with some sly maneuvering, she discovered one of his associates had indeed 'bought' her for $80,000 US. Her husband needed $100,000 US to help pay off his younger brother's gambling debts back in Beijing. At the time, she was 3 months' pregnant with her husband's baby.

In desperation she sought the help of another Chinese man, the head of a smuggling ring. He, together with four other men, got Li Hua back to China and then kept her in a countryside location while trying to extort money from her family. While her family was trying to get the several thousands of dollars together, she began to hemorrhage. The men sent her back to her home, but it was too late. She had lost her baby. Only at this point in her story-telling did Li Hua begin to cry. She paused but continued her story, now more animated than when we began. She then divorced her husband. He returned to Beijing and harassed her with threatening phone calls, obscene letters, and embarrassing accusations in front of her neighbors. Losing face with her neighbors was Li Hua's greatest concern.

During the 4 months since her return to Beijing, she had become increasingly frightened of strangers and refused to stay alone. Because of her troubled sleep and auditory hallucinations, her family took her to a general hospital; the doctor there recommended her admission to a psychiatric hospital.

I was even more intrigued. Was this fantastic story true or was it part of a very complex and grandiose delusional scheme? No information about it was recorded in her medical record, and none of the hospital staff knew anything about it. If it were true, it was obvious to me the woman was suffering from posttraumatic stress disorder (PTSD) rather than schizophrenia.

My interpreter and I were able to confirm with family members that her story was true. In four more sessions, I taught her and a friend who visited daily about PTSD. I reassured Li Hua that anyone experiencing the things she had would have similar symptoms of nightmares and hallucinations. These were not signs of her losing her sanity. I taught her how to stop the internal voices she was hearing, and we also worked out a plan of desensitization to men, so her fear of them gradually receded.

Her transformation was like the unfolding of a rose. By the end of a 1-month hospitalization, she was smiling, relaxed, and free of the symptoms that had brought her to the hospital. My interpreter, a Chinese nurse who had never witnessed the power of a therapeutic relationship, was convinced that our interventions, rather than medication, affected the positive change. I am not sure the other staff would agree. Her diagnoses and medication regime were unchanged. But I know, beyond a doubt, what made a big difference in this Chinese woman's life. ∎

Marlys Bueber, MN, RN, CNS
1995

READERS IN
NEED

Once a nurse, always a nurse.

I have learned the truth of this adage many times over during the last 14 years. That's how long it's been since I have done any clinical nursing. I thought I had left the field for good in 1984 when I was hired as a feature writer at a daily newspaper. I was burned out on nursing when I applied for the job, so I made no mention of my previous career when I interviewed with the editor.

After a couple of years of writing general features, however, I found myself peeking over the shoulder of the medical reporter who sat next to me. When she left the paper for another job, I applied for her position. Asked what my credentials were, I confessed that I had been a registered nurse for 15 years. I told no one else, but the word got around, and suddenly I had coworkers and staff from other departments standing at my desk for advice.

The questions were varied. Could you look at this rash? My father is getting forgetful—what should we do? Should I be concerned about this vaginal infection I've had for a month? Do you know a good endocrinologist? Do you think my blood pressure

medicine could be causing me to be dizzy?

I also began to hear from readers. They would see a story I had written about a particular disease or new treatment and call me, sometimes to get further information, sometimes to tell me of their problems. Often they just wanted a sympathetic ear. I had to learn to be part nurse, part psychologist, part social worker. Sometimes helping others interfered with my real job, but I could never turn down a request for help.

I remember a couple of calls especially well. One was from the mother of a reporter who had left for another job out of state. The woman, in her early 50s, had recently been diagnosed with colon cancer. She had no health insurance and could not afford further medical care. She had tried to apply for Medi-Cal, but had been told that her income was a few dollars too high to qualify. When she related these problems to her son, who was in Texas, he said he didn't know what to do, "'but call E'Louise. She'll know."

When the woman told me this, I was worried that I could not live up to such an expectation. Fortunately, I had developed a nice fat Rolodex filled with sources and experts in the medical industry. I called a contact at a community clinic whom I knew to be adept at 'tweaking' the rules of Medi-Cal in order to help the truly needy. She told me she would help. I was so relieved, so grateful, and felt as though I had really made a difference, even though I never met my caller.

On another occasion, a worried mother called me one morning after reading my story about bee sting allergies. Her 7-year-old son's bee sting kit had expired. She was worried because the pharmacist had refused to give her another, citing some obscure recent changes in Medi-Cal rules. The mother was afraid to let her son attend school because there had been a problem with bees swarming on the playground.

It took 3 hours of phone calls and explanations with the pharmacist, the school, and the Medi-Cal bureaucracy before the mother was finally able to obtain the kit for her son. I was a little peeved that she even had me arranging a ride to the pharmacy for her, but I couldn't stand the thought of her second-grader missing days of school because of government red tape.

There have been many other times when people in need have called, sent me an E-mail, come to my desk, or stopped me in the employee lounge. Sometimes their requests begin with, "You don't know me, but I heard you're a nurse and I wonder if you knew . . ."

I once joked that if I had a nickel for every piece of medical advice I'd given, I'd be a well-paid journalist. The next morning I arrived at work to find a message floating across my computer's screen saver—Medical Advice: 5 cents. ∎

E'Louise Ondash, RN
1984-1998

132

MRS. LONG

Six months into training at nursing school, the instructors decide whether you will be successful as a nurse. In my program, many students were eliminated because of poor grades. Those who were not cut went on to receive their nursing cap. In 1954, I was almost dropped before capping. For me, it was not anatomy and physiology or microbiology; my grades were fine. Nevertheless, I received the dreaded call to meet with the director of the nursing school. I was on probation because I didn't communicate with the patients.

Tearful but determined, I asked my friends "How do you talk to patients?" The best advice offered to me was to ask the patients about their family. Everyone likes to talk about their families. I figured I could do that.

The very next day, I was giving a bed bath to an elderly man. Under the drawn cubicle curtains, I saw the white stockings and shoes of my instructor, Mrs. Long, approaching. Quickly, I asked the man about his family. Suddenly, I was met with a torrent of sobs and tears. It seems he had only recently lost his wife. I was devastated and felt like the world's worst nurse. I had caused the poor man such sadness.

I don't remember completing his bath. I was too busy comforting him—that came naturally. Mrs. Long was delighted. Somehow, I established rapport with the patient and encouraged him to vent his pain, or so she thought.

I went on from there, hopefully, not making too many patients cry. I found that with practice, I really could talk to patients. When I graduated, one of my favorite instructors told me, "I don't know what you'll ever do for nursing, but nursing has done wonders for you." ∎

Barbara Fendorak, RN
1954

BILLY

Billy Holland was a tall, gangly 21-year-old guy from the inner city, admitted frequently to our chronic psych ward. He had a diagnosis of schizophrenia and often was violent and aggressive. Whenever his behavior was violent, he would be restrained by guards. If the behavior was repeated frequently, he would be sent to the psychiatric prison facility for the criminally insane. Billy was terrified of this place and would cry and wail painfully when being transferred. He reported abusive treatment by both guards and other inmates. When he was violent, the staff would tell him he would be sent to the prison, but this did not influence his behavior. He did not seem to be able to control his violence, even with the help of antipsychotic medications.

Working as a psychiatric CNS, I was distressed whenever Billy was sent to the downstate psychiatric prison. He was such an appealing and friendly person when he was not violent and I liked him. One day I decided to talk to him about controlling his violent behavior. I

Jacquelyn H. Flaskerud, PhD, RN, FAAN

asked if he could tell me if he thought he could not control himself. He asked what would happen if he thought he could not control himself. I told him, "We'll help you."

"Are you strong, Jackie?" he asked. I thought a minute and then said "Yes." "Strong as a bull, right?" Again I hesitated and then nodded. He squeezed my biceps muscle and then said "Yep, strong as a bull." I was more than a little embarrassed with this description, as I've never had muscle strength and was actually a great deal smaller than Billy. Every day Billy would ask me if I was strong, and then he would squeeze my biceps and I would agree that I was strong as a bull. The ward lost its tension for a couple of weeks as Billy laughed and talked and helped out with other patients, occasionally shouting out "Are you strong, Jackie?" During this time, he gave us the gift of joy, spirit, and friendship.

I went away for 2 weeks and when I came back Billy had been sent downstate again. We didn't see him for a year. Finally, we heard that he had died while at the downstate facility. His mother came later to pick up some of his things and she confirmed his death. She said he was troubled and afraid and "maybe it was for the best." She thought he died of heart failure. We all wondered and missed him. I know I was able to influence him in his time with us; he has continued to influence me. ∎

ROBERT

Robert was an emergency admission as a result of postelectric shock and burns sustained while on his job earlier in the day. During report, his light went on. "He wants his pain medication," the charge nurse said.

I was a relatively new RN on this med/surg unit. After receiving our assignments, I began my rounds, a little anxious about the first patient encounter of the evening. This particular evening, my anxiety was worse since I had been off for several days. I hesitantly approached room 326E, and there inside was Robert, a 36-year-old married electrician.

Robert was alone. His eyes were attentive and intense and he looked afraid. He didn't volunteer to speak. Robert's hands were wrapped in gauze dressings and elevated on a pillow. He did not move, and his respirations were slow and shallow—I remember staring for a moment to make sure he was breathing. All he said was "The pain is too much. Can you help me?" I assured him that I would get him a shot immediately. Robert was a 'good' patient. He never refused anything, and he never asked for anything, except his pain medication. He seemed to always be in pain.

Robert was assigned to my care for the duration of his hospitalization. The primary task of the shift

was to redress his wounds and assess his hand and finger range of motion during the process. It was an awesome, painful, and time-consuming process, requiring mutual trust, sensitivity, and patience for both of us. Most of all, we both had to face and conquer our fears, which were never openly discussed. I did not tell Robert that I had never seen this type of wound before and that it was difficult for me to see him in such pain.

Dressing changes were done after visiting hours every night at 8:00 pm. I would give Robert his medication 20 minutes beforehand. Then, before his wife and visitors left, I would begin some mental preparation with Robert and his visitors. We would talk superficially about how things were going and other casual, social topics. Initially, Robert would never participate. He did not want the radio or television on and would not allow the curtains between him and his roommate to be opened. He would sit in bed watching our interactions—attentive but removed.

A few days passed before he gradually began to connect with the staff and his visitors. Our plan was to set the television and radio at the lowest volume to serve as a helpful distraction. A week went by before he initiated conversation. He said he was afraid and then he started to cry. He feared rejection, pain, and paralysis, and he felt out of control of everything, especially his life and his future.

The staff worked together on helping him regain control of his situation. His pain medication was ordered at set times, and other therapies and medications were offered as needed. We explored together the extent of the damage and the progress his hands and fingers were making each day.

Robert's wife was supportive of him but equally fearful. Although she was present during most of the daytime hours, she would not participate in the evening dressing changes. She too was working through her losses. Robert understood his wife's behavior. He said that he preferred her to rest peacefully rather than be tormented by 'this awful sight' before going to sleep.

By day 10, his oversized charred hands and fingers, covered with Silvadene cream and gauze, were taking a more recognizable human shape. When Robert was able to voluntarily flex his digits, ever so slightly, he laughed a hearty but nervous laugh. His spirit grew stronger each day. He focused his attention and energy on getting through this debridement phase so he could go home.

Robert became more receptive to using his imagination to help him through each step of his hospitalization, and especially his interactions with the plastic surgeons and physical therapists. We used prayer,

imagery, therapeutic touch, visualization, and music to enhance his awareness of and faith in his progress. He was a quick learner and a good student.

Robert's progress was continuous, and he began sharing the vision he had of starting a family and getting back to work. By his 8th week of hospitalization, Robert was prepared for discharge with a plan for outpatient physical therapy and rehabilitation. His dressings would be changed after whirlpool treatments and an exercise regimen.

The night before his discharge, I wished him my best before the end of my shift. I had grown attached to Robert. He was excited about going home. As weeks passed, Robert's name faded from daily conversation. But I missed him and wondered about him.

A month later, I was in the hospital parking lot when I saw Robert and his wife heading for his daily treatment. He told me that he was down to one treatment a day and experiencing very little pain. They were both looking forward to their future together. Robert hugged me and thanked me again for being there for him even when he wasn't at his best. His wife thanked me for being there when she needed to talk.

Long after we parted, I felt thrilled at his progress and a sense of personal fullfillment for having touched their lives. I believe I made a difference in Robert's life because I cared. ∎

Santa J. Crisall, MA, RN, C
1979

MARGARET

I had not been in my job very long when I was visited by a young woman, an outpatient surgery nurse who was glad I was here, because "oncology nurses here don't know anything about psychological support for patients who have cancer." Margaret had had breast cancer, and only by seeking resources in her home town and identifying a supportive breast center nurse had she been able to receive the care she needed to get through her chemotherapy. She was very angry that this had not been available. I was very surprised at her interpretation of oncology nurses, because as an oncology CNS for more than 12 years, I felt that psychosocial support was our strong point! However, I managed to hold my counsel and let her vent.

I discovered that Margaret volunteered for the American Cancer Society, and counseled and supported other women who had breast cancer and had undergone mastectomy. I served on an American Cancer Society committee with her and found her insights invaluable. But one day when I went to a committee meeting, it was announced that Margaret was resigning from the committee to spend more time on the

Mary Ann Bord-Hoffman, MN, MA, RN, AOCN
1993

pursuits that were important to her. She was thinking of going back to interior design school. While I felt disappointed, because I knew the contribution she made as a nurse, I also realized that sometimes it is important for a person who has cancer to distance oneself from it.

That year the hospital honored its first "cancer survivor" as part of the American Cancer Society Survivors' celebration. Margaret was the first so named. Not long afterwards, she identified a wish to establish a cancer resource center for patients and their families at the hospital.

Margaret, even after leaving nursing, still seemed to show up in patients' rooms and in my office for various projects she wanted to undertake. I never pushed her to continue, but felt that my role was to be supportive of what she wanted. Eventually, she was able to say that she wanted to work in an expanded nursing role, helping women with breast cancer. We discussed various options and the requirements for each of these. One day Margaret came to my office and told me: "I am going back to school to get my BSN. I want to be a CNS like you." Something I had done had contributed to this marvelous young woman deciding to pursue a career in oncology nursing. Margaret is in the process of completing her masters in nursing, fulfilling her dream. Every time I recall this, I am joyful for those patients and for my nursing profession. In this case, it is hard to tell which of us was more touched by a nurse. ∎

WILLIAM
AND MARI

As the program coordinator for the hospital's geriatric hip fracture program, I have the opportunity to meet a variety of patients and families. As nurses, we all know that sometimes we may be touched by personal issues.

I had the opportunity meet a Russian family. The patient, William, was a 72-year-old man who lived at home with his wife, Mari. His hip was fractured when he slid off a kitchen chair. His medical history included dementia—Alzheimer type—and chronic lymphocytic leukemia. Talking with his wife through an interpreter, I learned that he had been sick a few days before the fall. Mari had been the primary caregiver for 4 years.

I watched the interactions between Mari and her husband's daughter during the orthopedic physician's visit. They did not look at or talk to one another. Mari asked the physician very important questions. Among these, she asked whether William would walk on his own after the operation. Mari further explained that due to her husband's condition, she needed to assist him and encourage him to walk. The physician answered, "He will, with assistance

and rehabilitation." Her husband's daughter commented, "It was a shame that he fell."

In my responsibility as program coordinator, I made daily rounds to see how the patients and their families were progressing. One day, Mari asked me if I had a few minutes to talk with her. She told me her story.

Mari grew up in Russia, married, and had a daughter. After her first husband died, she took a job as a seamstress. She came over to the United States to be a housekeeper for William's family. William was a holocaust survivor and had emigrated from Russia years before.

During her first year, while Mari was working for William's family, William's wife died suddenly from a heart attack. A year later, Mari and William fell in love and were married. William's health declined over time, however, and at times Mari began feeling like his personal nurse. She said that she only slept a few hours each night out of her concern for William's safety during his periods of confusion. Mari cried, saying that she had tried hard to love his daughter, but that the daughter just did not seem to care or even want to talk with her. She would visit them only when she needed money. Then Mari said something that still echoes in my mind. "Life is like a history book—you can't change what has happened in a person's life, you can only accept it and do the best you can."

I wonder how many of us deal with similar situations, trying to change things bound by past history that we are powerless to change? ∎

Susan M. Leininger, MSN, RN
1998

HARRY

The call came from the medical ICU. "We have an 87-year-old gentleman here, admitted in DKA." Harry had no prior history of diabetes, was admitted with a blood sugar greater than 1400, and a new diagnosis of Type I diabetes. Furthermore, he was confused, and a psych consult had been ordered. And Harry lived alone!

Where should I begin to teach this man all he'd need to know to control his diabetes? This was going to be a major-league challenge.

In the MICU, I only visited Harry briefly, just so he'd recognize me when I started in full force. Two days later, Harry was transferred to 6D medical floor, and I started the formidable task of teaching him survival skills. If he were to continue living alone, at the very least, he would need basic diet knowledge, the dexterity to prepare and administer insulin and test his blood sugar, and the ability to recognize and treat hypoglycemia.

He had been seen briefly by a dietitian, so I decided to start by assessing what he knew and reinforcing what he had been taught. I first asked him if he ate breakfast (this would be an important meal since he would be taking insulin). "Oh yes, I

make oatmeal every morning" he said. "Great!" I replied, "and how about lunch?" "Well, lunch will be a problem because I don't eat until 2 o'clock."

I figured he probably slept late, and, if breakfast wasn't until 10 am, a 2-o'clock lunch was fine. So, the next logical question was "Well, what time do you eat your oatmeal?" The answer, "Four o'clock in the morning." My reply, "Why on earth do you eat your breakfast so early?" His response, "Well, I have to leave for work at 5 am!"

Later on, I was ready to start teaching him to prepare insulin. I said "Harry, you'll need to learn to use a syringe. I know you live alone, but is there someone who can bring in your glasses from home?" His answer, "I don't wear glasses!"

A few days and several visits later, Harry left the hospital, no longer confused, and ready to take on his new life with diabetes. He would be fixing his insulin twice a day and was very clear which dose was which, and he would be testing his blood sugar several times a day. And he would go back to work, but he'd take a break for a mid-morning snack.

So often, when we see a person's ability to function compromised by an acute phase of illness or a new diagnosis, we tend to forget that that same person has "another life" that may be quite active and productive.

I learned from Harry and was inspired by him to look at the whole person, which is often a pleasant surprise. ■

Mary Loftus, BSN, RN, CDE
1998

SUSAN

"We need you to come in to see this suicidal patient. The sheriff took a gun away from her. She's being very uncooperative." It was 1 am, and I had just been called to one of the emergency departments that was served by our hospital-based psychiatric evaluation and triage team.

No matter how many patients I evaluate who are in crisis, the experience is different each time. In order to make that interpersonal connection, I always look for some way to understand the feelings behind the 'chaos.'

"Yes, I'm Susan. What do you want? No one believes me. Why should I talk to you? I don't want to kill myself. They won't let me leave. I can't even find out about my daughter." I was hit by a barrage of angry words and some hysteria from this slight, gown-clad, 30ish woman who was propping herself up on the gurney in a stance of defiance and desperation. Her impatience changed to tears as I stood there quietly listening. Perhaps that's the connection? I encouraged Susan to tell me why she was worried.

She and her family were staying at a local motel so Susan could have

Margo Foltz Wilson, MS, RN, CS, CGP
1997

surgery by a local doctor. During a heated argument with her husband over her daughter missing a curfew, she had pulled the gun. She assured me it was only to make her husband realize she was upset. She admitted to me that she had made some poor choices in men, and she didn't want this to happen to her daughter.

The gun story was confusing. Susan carried it for protection after being raped a few years ago. The sheriff decided it was a domestic squabble but wanted Susan evaluated to be sure she was not going to hurt herself or someone else. Paramedics thought she had threatened to shoot herself.

I did a thorough lethality assessment: no previous suicide attempts, no psychiatric history, not even any current drug or alcohol use, no immediate intent or plan, but Susan was certainly impulsive. Her current husband was in the waiting room and told me a similar story, verifying my impression. Susan was not suicidal.

As I talked to Susan about seeking some counseling for herself and her family, she took my hand. "Thank you for believing me. I was scared no one would. I've learned a lesson."

Later, I remembered my frustration as a student nurse trying to learn how to deal with patients whose behaviors were puzzling. Now as a seasoned clinical specialist, I still marvel at the simplicity of our art: finding the universality of the feelings the patient and I share. ■

JERRY

The intermediate care unit at our hospital cares for more stable patients than usually would be in the ICU. It was difficult to hear the ventilator alarms in this setting, so we had a central alarm system to alert us to all ventilator problems. Jerry was a 35-year-old trauma victim who had suffered a broken neck in a fall from a roof. The fracture was high in the spinal cord. Jerry couldn't breathe at all without the ventilator. When he first came to us, he was unconscious. The physicians thought that at the time of the fall he had been without the ability to breathe and suffered permanent brain damage. My instinct told me that he heard and understood.

Indeed, after several weeks, he did wake up and was able to communicate with us: first with blinks and eventually by mouthing words. But he never regained any movement below the neck and relied on his caregivers for everything. I was his primary nurse; I worked with him every day and got to know him and his family very well. In time, he became strong enough to use a talking tracheotomy tube. This bedside device allows diversion of air through the patient's voice box so he can speak.

One day, I was in the kitchen getting ice chips for Jerry, and I heard the ventilator alarm. I hurried the few feet necessary to see which ventilator was alarming and saw that it was Jerry's. I knew he was alone and couldn't breathe without the ventilator. I rushed to his room to give him breaths using the manual bag. As he regained consciousness, I hooked him back up to the ventilator. He was frantic to talk to me, so I occluded the valve to allow him to speak. His terrified eyes were filled with tears as he struggled to tell me what had happened. He heard the ventilator alarm and knew that he must have become disconnected. "I began to fall into a deep, dark tunnel. I called your name, over and over. I knew you were the only one who could bring me back" he sobbed. "Then I started coming back, like you were pulling me out of the tunnel, and I could hear you calling me."

I'm not sure what I believe about out-of-body experiences. Who can decipher the spiritual from the imagined? It doesn't really matter. For me, the image that Jerry drew is a representation of all the hours I had spent with him, the trust we had built, his ultimate dependence on his caregivers—and especially his primary nurse. This bond is real. The person-to-person engagement is the essence of the bond. Our ability to touch the souls of others makes our work and our lives worthwhile. ∎

Sharon Henchal Deeny, MSN, RN, CCRN
1989

MR.
HIGGINS

I think it was Melody Chenevert who said that nursing is a career measured in moments, not in years. And it is true. Moments...and faces. I can close my eyes and see so many faces. The names, for the most part, have long been forgotten, but the faces remain.

It began when I was a student nurse. Mercy Hospital is where I became a nurse. There are always patients in your training whom you remember, celebrate, mourn, for reasons too numerous to count. I can still remember, will always remember, Mr. Higgins, a gentleman whose colostomy 'exploded' after he was erroneously given a very harsh cathartic in preparation for some kind of test he was to have the following day. The 'prep' was not intended for someone with a colostomy, and the result was disastrous.

I was a freshman nursing student, 18 years old. Mr. Higgins was *my* patient, committed to *my* care, and, as we stood in the bathroom that evening covered with feces, with bath towels covered with feces, he looked at me and said "I'm so sorry about this." I responded immediately, spontaneously, and truthfully by telling him it was "no problem." Even at that young age, as inexperienced as I was, I was able to empathize with him in a way that, I believe, only a nurse can. I could somehow feel what he felt...and it was not only my duty to help—I wanted to help. I cared about him, his situation, his life, and he felt it.

As we stood in the bathroom of that ward, we both began to laugh. Standing there, hardly able to bear the smell, we laughed and laughed. The comedy, the tragedy, the moment is what we shared. That incident was a revelation to me. I was not only surprised at myself, I was completely in awe of the process. The whole thing was, somehow, bigger than I was. It was what I read about, observed when I watched the 'experienced' nurses relate to patients. It was what I felt when one of my instructors told a patient's son to "get another opinion" when his father was not getting well or doing well, even though she jeopardized her own position by saying that. It was that connection nurses have with their patients, and patients have with their nurses. It was the beginning of a career of connections, moment by moment. ∎

Kelly Gaul, MSN, RN, CS
1972

MRS. JUDD

During the end-of-shift report, the staff described Mrs. Judd as emotional, a hypochondriac, and uncooperative. She had not followed postoperative instructions to lift her operative leg every 2 hours, had been weepy, and requested pain medication too often.

Mrs. Judd was an obese African American woman who had undergone knee surgery the previous day. She had told me she was "scared" and afraid of hospitals, needles, and medical procedures. The night before her surgery, I explained the surgical procedure, pre- and postoperative activities to expect, and taught her to practice tightening the thigh muscle and lifting her leg from the bed. Mrs. Judd and I seemed to have a special bond and my explanations were calming.

I talked with Mrs. Judd for a few minutes. She was extremely afraid that she would injure the surgery site if she either exercised the leg muscles or lifted the leg. Again, I reassured her that, although painful, the exercises would facilitate more rapid recovery. I reviewed the rehabilitation process and how important her contribution was during recovery. I gave her pain medication because it had been 3

Perri J. Bomar, PhD, RN
1969

hours since her last injection. After the medication had relieved her pain, I returned to her room to coach through the exercises.

Prior to surgery, she had became less anxious when I gently touched her hand. Repeating caring touch, this time on her leg, I very lightly placed my hand on her thigh and said to her "You can do this, close your eyes and concentrate on your leg where my hand is. Think how warm it is and tighten the muscles like you did for me a couple of nights ago. You can do it again."

As I laid my hand on her thigh, I silently prayed and continued to encourage her, "Contract, release, contract, release, lift your leg." After several times of such instruction, she lifted her leg about 3 inches off the bed and held it a few seconds. Her face turned from a frown and tears to a smile. She exclaimed "I did it!, I did it! You helped me. I couldn't have done this without you! Thank you so much." She repeated this exercise several more times that evening and was able to lift her leg higher each time.

The next evening, I saw Mrs. Judd walking down the hall with her husband. She was smiling and said to her husband as I passed, "That's my nurse. She taught me to practice my exercises and how to lift my leg so I could get up and start walking. I couldn't have done it without her." This was one of those special times that I was thankful to be a nurse and was able to assist someone to heal using care, pharmacology, prayer, and a holistic therapeutic technique. ∎

MARY

I was doing my annual "Managing
Holiday Stress" lecture on a cold
December evening one week in the
hospital auditorium. This lecture
has been traditionally part of our
behavioral health department's
holiday gift to the hospital and the
community. As a clinical nurse
specialist, I regularly presented on
wellness for the general public. One
never knows what one will 'get' at
these lectures. I had spent a fair
amount of time preparing for the
talk. The audience turnout was
dismal. Or so I thought.

I turned my back from the large
empty auditorium to collect my
things and leave. When I turned back
again to the seating, I was surprised
to see one woman, a senior citizen,
sitting alone in the middle of the
large room. "Oh my" she said in an
embarrassed tone. "No one else is
coming. Well, I won't take your
time." She began to gather her things
to leave. I thanked her for coming
and sat down near her. I asked,
"Why did you come here tonight?"
"I love these lectures" she replied. "I
don't go out at night except to come
to these talks. I don't really have a
reason to go out at night anymore. I
don't understand why more people
aren't here. I knew it would be
interesting."

"Well, how do you spend the
holidays?" I inquired, hoping that

I could help to make her venture
out in the cold worthwhile. "I
don't do Christmas, you know. I
don't have the money for gifts in
boxes. Today, everyone has
everything, anyway." I agreed and
asked if she'd like to do next
year's talk with me. She smiled
and we laughed.

"I've had to 'downsize' (her
word) and don't have room for lots
of stuff anymore" she said. "I've
been able to give away a lot this
season!" She sparkled as she said
this.

I commented that giving is part
of the holiday spirit. "Yes" she
replied. "That's mentioned in
Eastern religions, isn't it?"

"Oh yes" I answered. "And in the
prayer of St. Francis: 'It is in giving
that we receive.' "

"Oh, that is right, isn't it?" was
her cheerful reply. "Well," she went
on, "don't you think we should
practice that part of Christmas
every day?" I smiled and nodded.

I was wondering how she coped
with the holidays, so I asked, "What
do you do?"

She held her head humbly. "I
don't do Christmas. Instead, I go to
the soup kitchens downtown and
feed the homeless. I really enjoy
that. Thanksgiving is my favorite. I
have so much to be thankful for in
my life. I've always had food and
shelter."

I asked about family and friends,
in concern for her loneliness (I was
thinking about inviting her to a
potluck I was to attend later in the
evening).

144

"I have no family, but I have a few friends. Therefore, I don't like a lot of those family things. I'm not comfortable. All that food is more than I like and more than I need, as well." She continued, "Sometimes those gatherings can be like 'false tinsel,' just like the emphasis on presents that cost money. I see how that makes people crazy. I work weekends in a gift shop and watch people suffer over the perfect gift." She hesitated. "I think the whole gift thing can be kind of fake sometimes. You know, people with possessions are possessed." I nodded and asked permission to quote her. We laughed again. "You are so kind" she said. "Well, you know I've done all that Christmas gift stuff in the past. I have grey hair now." Her snow-white hair seemed to glow as she giggled and combed it with her fingers.

"I did go to Christmas in the Prado in Balboa Park. It was wonderful! The park was filled with children, music and beautiful sights. You really should go next year!" I assured her that I would.

I told her that I thought she had the spirit of the season, and that her giving and acknowledgment of others was what Christmas was about. She became coy, bowed her head, and repeated, "You are kind."

"You know, I think you really do 'do' Christmas," I insisted. To my surprise, this wise woman quietly replied "You really think I'm OK?"

I assured her that she was.

I asked her name. She replied "Mary."

I told her she had given me a gift.

I turned back to the stage to once again collect my things. When I turned back, Mary was no longer in the auditorium. I said "good-bye" ... to myself. ∎

Jim Kane, MN, RN, CS, CNAA
1992

MRS. DUNDEE

Mrs. Dundee was a 50-year-old woman with end-stage lung cancer that had metastasized to her brain and bones. She was from out-of-state, but she and her husband had done their homework and selected our university teaching hospital and our doctors. I'd spoken to Mr. Dundee twice while Mrs. Dundee was semiconscious and had established some rapport.

Family and friends from all over were gathering to say good-bye to the patient, including her daughter, who was 8 months' pregnant. The room was often filled with laughter and tears, and many loving stories of good times in the past.

I visited one day and was surprised to see the patient out of bed. I greeted Mrs. Dundee, and she began talking softly, her voice barely audible. Her friends began interpreting her statements to me, explaining that Mrs. Dundee was meaning this or that, and that she was confused. I continued to focus on the patient and encouraged Mrs. Dundee to speak. I also encouraged the family to listen to her.

Mrs. Dundee then told us an amazing story of sitting alone in her motor home soon after being diagnosed with cancer. She described crying her heart out, overcome with fear about the future. After a while she began talking to God, and soon felt a warm breeze move over her, followed by being completely filled with peace, a feeling that remained with her ever since. She said "Everything will be okay, I'm in God's hands. I'm so lucky to have my husband, I'm so lucky to have my family, I'm so lucky to have my friends" and she went on and on, listing people she cared about. She relaxed as she spoke, and her voice became stronger and clearer as we listened. A sense of awe descended on the room. When she became silent, I acknowledged the beautiful gift she'd given us. One of her friends offered to write the story down and share it with family and friends who had not been present

I believe it took a nurse to recognize the potential in this situation. This was a sacred moment in Mrs. D's life. She was displaying more energy and alertness than she had in several days. She had something to say. I modeled patience, presence, and active listening for the friends and family gathered, and this empowered her to bring forth her story. Once her story was received, its value became clear to all of us. Her daughter would write down her mother's words for those not present, including the unborn grandchild. Mrs. Dundee's story would live on. ■

Ramita Bonadonna, MSN, RN, CS
1997

OUR
PARTIAL
HOSPITAL
PATIENTS

One of the skills a psychiatric nurse must possess is the ability to act as a buffer between our patients and the world in general, and to help them integrate as inconspicuously as possible into the mainstream. This is not always easy. Those of us in the field are there because we respect, and often love, the patients. We understand the struggles people with serious mental illness go through to just 'stay afloat.' The general public is often ignorant of the difficulties these patients face.

Several years ago, I took a group of patients to a Padres game. In addition to nine patients, another staff person accompanied me. Outings of this type were considered therapeutic in assisting outpatients to better acclimate to the public at large. As we sat down in the stadium, one young man became very agitated because he believed the blimp floating overhead was sending messages to the crowd about his sexual preferences. After talking with him for several minutes, trying to reassure him this was not accurate, the woman next to me interrupted us to wonder if there was life on

Mars. She continued to become increasingly upset and wonder if the next ice age might start while the game was on "and what will we do if there are glaciers in the parking lot?" Again I spent time reassuring, explaining, and encouraging her to focus on the activity on the playing field.

A female patient from New York began to ask questions about the game. This was short-lived, though, as she quickly moved on, talking about her personal issues, and had to be restrained from such public airing of personal problems. Meanwhile, I became aware of a strong smell of marijuana. It seems the left-field bleachers were known for sunning and smoking. The other staff member and myself had to be alert for any attempts on the part of our folks to join in.

At the large food court, one female patient became upset because she thought we had left her behind. I came upon her as she was crying and calling out for us. As I approached, so did a bystander. This man began to taunt our patient saying "Are you crazy? You're out of control." She continued to cry and then began to yell back. By now we had a crowd of about 50 people watching. He continued to taunt our patient. I continued to try to get the man to be quiet and tried to take our patient to our van. He was not to be deterred. It was at least 5 more minutes (and seemed like 5 years) before the man backed off and I was able to drag our patient away. This entire time I reassured the assembled crowd that I was in 'control' and they need not be concerned. I then spent much time reassuring the patient that her behavior was not nearly as inappropriate as the so-called 'healthy' bystander.

Several innings later, three well-dressed young men came in and sat down in front of us. Soon they stood up, took off their coats, shirts, and ties, and proceeded to cut them up (I had heard that the latest fad was to get clothes from a thrift store and then destroy them in public). I sat there, amazed at this display. I was equally amazed to discover that the patients paid absolutely no attention.

When we returned to the hospital, other staff members asked how I enjoyed the game and who had won? Having my memory filled with Martians, glaciers, blimps, men cutting their clothes off, skirmishes, and pot, I could only reply "What game?" ∎

Gale Osborn, MA, RN, C
1976

MR. GORDON

I was seeing patients in the office with my new colleague, Dr. Frankl. As a new clinical nurse specialist, fresh out of my masters program, I was unsure about my role. In spite of this, I saw Dr. Frankl's patients, listened to their symptoms, conducted physical exams, and added a good measure of patient teaching and counseling to each visit.

At the end of my morning, I entered the exam room of my last patient, a 44-year-old man who had an abnormal electrocardiogram and chest pain with exertion. I had not seen this patient before, but his record indicated that he had had coronary artery bypass surgery 2 years prior. Now he was back with indications that he needed more treatment. I consulted with Dr. Frankl, who told me that he had taken care of this patient for several years, trying to get him to take care of himself, but to no avail. He said bluntly: "Mr. Gordon is a drinker. Further therapy is not an option if he keeps on drinking." My mission was clear.

I reentered the room and sat down with Mr. Gordon. My news was no surprise to him—the combination of his electrocardiogram and his symptoms suggested that his coronary artery disease had returned. And, Dr. Frankl said that he needed to quit drinking if he was going to be a candidate for a repeat operation. What I said next, however, was a surprise to both of us. I told him "You have to quit drinking and I'm going to help you. And, we need to do this immediately. I don't want to take any chances that you could have a heart attack while you're getting ready to quit!"

He was astounded! And tears came to his eyes. We began to talk about his prior attempts to quit drinking, thoughts concerning a plan for quitting, and the expected response from his family. His wife was divorcing him because of his drinking, so he didn't think that she would be of much support. We agreed upon inpatient treatment and Alcoholics Anonymous for later support.

I sent Mr. Gordon home to pack a bag while I made arrangements for him to be admitted to an alcohol treatment facility. He was to return by 1:00 pm to learn about the arrangements. 1:00 pm came and went and Mr. Gordon did not return. 1:30 pm passed. And, at about 2:15 pm, in walked Mr. Gordon with his packed bag. I put him in a cab and sent him to the alcohol treatment facility. I visited him every other day.

I knew absolutely nothing about helping an alcoholic stop drinking. So, I made appointments with local experts and visited treatment facilities to learn as much as I could about the treatment of alcoholism. It was then that I understood how naive my approach had been.

After 3 weeks of inpatient care, Mr. Gordon was discharged home. He connected with Alcoholics Anonymous and visited me at weekly intervals. Dr. Frankl referred him for reoperation and he underwent a second successful coronary artery bypass surgery about 2 months after our initial meeting.

Although I didn't see Mr. Gordon for years after that, he stayed in my mind intermittently. I never knew what it was about this situation or our interaction that had allowed me to gain his trust and his confidence so quickly. Why did he allow me to reach out and pull him in, when quite obviously, others (his wife, Dr. Frankl) had tried and failed?

About 2 years ago (almost 14 years later), I received a call from the hospital operator saying that there was a Mr. Gordon in Room 643 who was looking for me. I no longer saw patients as a clinical nurse specialist—I was a clinical researcher now—so it was unusual for a patient to ask for me. But, the name sounded familiar. I went to Room 643 just in time to see my former patient before he was discharged from the hospital.

I knew him the minute I saw him. He looked the same but a bit older and wiser. There was a woman with him whom he introduced as his new wife. He told me that he had seen my name on an office door and had tracked me down because he wanted to thank me for all I had done for him. We both held back tears as he told his wife "This is Barbara! I've talked about her for so many years and now you can finally meet her!" [And then to me] "You believed in me." ∎

Barbara Riegel, DNSc, RN, CS, FAAN
1983

FRED

Fred was middle-aged and had been very ill before having his surgery. Following surgery, Fred had many complications. He started to bleed internally around his heart several times after his initial surgery. Over a period of several weeks Fred developed other problems. Every new problem challenged the medical team to respond aggressively to give Fred the best chance in an increasingly uphill battle.

Fred never truly awakened from his surgery. He had a breathing tube inserted into his windpipe and was connected to a ventilator. Fred's family was struggling with not being able to have him talk with them. They were looking for some sense of stability. The nursing staff provided as much support as we could to them, answering questions, listening to fears.

Christmas Day arrived. Fred's morning lab work was abnormal; he needed numerous intravenous potassium and magnesium supplements. His vital signs indicated that Fred's battle might be coming to an end.

When the physicians made their rounds, I told them about Fred's lab work and about his mildly unstable vital signs. I asked how much potassium and magnesium they wanted to give Fred, and their reply took me completely by surprise. "We're not going to treat him this time. I think its best if we just let him go." With that the medical team was off to the next patient.

I looked at Fred, at the monitors and tubes coming from his chest and mouth. I thought about the incurable infection inside his chest wall. I thought about his family. I thought about Christmas Day. I thought about arbitrarily deciding this is the day we aren't going to treat him, anymore. Those words hit me again, "I think it's best if we just let him go." I decided to approach the team of doctors. "I think we need to treat Fred today," I said to them. They replied "No matter what we do, Fred isn't going to survive." "I know he's going to die, but not today," I insisted. "Not on Christmas Day." I was upset. "You can't just let this man go today. I don't care what we have to do to keep him alive, but he can't die on Christmas Day. How would you like to live the rest of your life knowing your husband or father died on Christmas Day?"

The team of doctors looked at me, and treated Fred. His family came on that day to visit, never knowing that a nurse forestalled the inevitable. They were able to spend Christmas together. The next day, with his family by his side, Fred died peacefully, surrounded by love. ∎

James P. Veronesi, MSN, RN, CEN

RUTH

I first met Ruth in 1980. She returned to the oncology clinic because a metastatic scalp lesion had been discovered by her dermatologist. The year before, she had undergone surgery and radiation therapy for breast cancer. Ruth had hoped that would be the end of it.

The outcome of the diagnostic work-up revealed a very advanced metastasis. The right lobe of her liver was completely obliterated by tumor. Her skeleton had 'hot spots' from top to bottom. Ruth was tearful as she agreed to participate in an investigational research study, although she never believed that the 'little white pill' was powerful enough to arrest her cancer. Sure enough, within 3 weeks, her repeat scans revealed a progression of the disease. The chemotherapy was immediately changed to a more conventional regimen including intravenous medications.

During this same time, I witnessed an amazing transformation of this meek and fragile woman. Ruth decided that she was not ready to die and that she wanted to actively participate in recovering her health. She converted to a vegetarian diet, began to walk a

mile each day despite the weather, and she began to swim twice a week. Most importantly, Ruth began to meditate twice daily. She used all of her imaginative skills to visualize her body working in partnership with the chemotherapy to eliminate the cancer cells. Ruth also initiated communication with her estranged daughter.

Ruth's liver scan began to fill in with normal, healthy tissue. The change was so dramatic that the nuclear medicine physician had to interpret it as normal. Initially he had thought that the name had been mislabeled. The 'hot spots' on the skeletal scan began to calcify. Clearly a healing was taking place on an emotional, spiritual and physical level...what a generous gift from God!

Ruth's disease stabilized for 13 months, until it returned with a vengeance. During this precious time she reconnected with her daughter and grandchildren. She learned how to express her needs in an assertive manner. She gained a heightened sensitivity of her spiritual being and she came to understand how blessed her life had been. Ruth had come to view the cancer as a gift.

My work now focuses on mind/body medicine, and I always use Ruth's experience to offer hope and inspiration to those in need. Although many years have passed since our meeting, Ruth's presence remains close to my heart. Knowing her has enhanced the quality of my life and my nursing career. ∎

Kathleen Krebs, BSN, RN
1980

LUCAS

Lucas was 9 months old when he came to our pediatric unit. I entered his room with trepidation. Was I really ready for this? My step was noiseless in my well-worn shoes, but the tiny, motionless form in the crib in front of me seemed to sense my presence. Almost imperceptibly, he tensed every muscle in his little body, preparing silently for an assault.

Lucas was the youngest child in a highly distressed family. A terrible domestic accident left him with severe burns over large portions of his torso, arms, and face. He had just spent several months in a regional burn center, where he had undergone extensive and painful treatment. He was transferred to our unit so that he could once again be near his family while at the same time continuing intensive physical therapy.

A first meeting with Lucas brought everyone to the same horrible conclusion. "He seems like a caged animal." He willingly allowed no one to touch him. His cries were precipitated simply by the presence of another human being. He did not respond to toys or efforts to play or interact, even from a distance.

Lucas stayed with us for 6 months. The most powerful memory I have of Lucas is of the day he finally returned home to his family. A chubby little toddler, walking gleefully from one of us to another, accepting gifts of toys and food from each and every willing giver. His smile was radiant and his giggle infectious.

His physical scars had been addressed by the miracles of modern medicine and would, we believed, with good follow-up eventually be relatively inconsequential. But the far deeper scars were healed by the love and attention he was able to experience from those caring for him in this unlikely setting. The patience and consistency in his daily routine helped him regain comfort and develop trust in human contact. ■

This event occurred while I was on active duty with the U.S. Army Nurse Corps, 1984. This work represents the views of the author and not necessarily those of the Army Medical Department, Department of the Army, or the Department of Defense.

Margaret Nelson, MSN, RN
1984

PATRICIA

Patricia, an Oglala Sioux woman, came in dressed in work clothes, smelling of cigarette smoke and sweat. Her brow was set and her eyes were steely hard and demanding, "I need pain medicine, are you the new doc?" I said I was the new health care provider, a nurse practitioner hired to provide primary care to the region's urban Indian community. "Well," she stated, "I need my medicine they always used to give me, my stomach hurts." She sat clutching her pelvis.

Patricia's chart revealed walk-in visits for relief of abdominal pain. The previous medical provider's pain medication was her sole treatment for more than a year.

After my examination, I offered Patricia an "energy healing" for her pain (a description I use to introduce therapeutic touch [TT] into a first-time visit). She agreed. Hand-scanning field assessment revealed to me that she was disconnected and out of balance. Her pain went beyond this particular pain experience. Over the pelvic region, I intuited a deep loss within her as if a major part of her was missing. Her pain subsided to a dull ache within minutes of beginning the first treatment. I suggested a diagnostic and treatment plan of both traditional and alternative medicine.

Subsequent visits with Patricia led to ongoing TT, and participation in a weekly women's spiritual "talking circle." Concurrently, I compiled an extensive medical records search from many other Indian Health Service (IHS) clinics she had attended over the years. They revealed exploratory operative reports, all normal for physical pathology. Yet the pain persisted. Eventually she became untrusting of health care systems and their providers.

Patricia had left a homogenous and multigenerational family environment to live in an urban space among strangers of many races. She, like many of the Indian clients, was labeled by dominant society members as mentally slow, uncooperative, and lazy. In her opinion, this stigmatization seemed to exude from previous health care providers and served to create what *she* perceived as a noncaring attitude. Patricia continued to have transient pain and I sent her to a gynecologist. The morning of her laparoscopy, I performed TT, taped her medicine bag onto her upper back, and prayed for either a diagnosis or an end to the pain. The study was negative. However, her pain never returned. She returned for TT and the talking circle. At each meeting, she revealed more of herself.

During a subsequent visit, Patricia revealed a clue to her long-time pain pattern, telling a story long held within. I recalled what I had detected on her initial TT scan—deep loss, a major missing part of her. Eight years before, on the reservation, Patricia's female relatives insisted she have a tubal ligation after her third child was born. Patricia suffered from alco-

154

holism. Although she did not really want the surgery that would take away her chances of future children, she gave in to her elders' pressure.

The child, Stacy, a beautiful little girl, captured Patricia's heart. This was a new beginning for her to stay clean and sober and to do something with her life. She was the best mother she could be to little Stacy.

At 6 months of age, Stacy contracted a respiratory infection. Community health workers on the reservation advised visiting the clinic. Patricia made three visits in 1 week. Each time, the physician told her "There is nothing wrong with the child...just a cold." Each visit she asserted her fears and asked him to do something. Patricia said he appeared hostile, uncaring, and specifically offended that she would suggest knowing more of her child's condition that he did.

He may have been acting in a caring manner acceptable in the dominant society. However, this reservation woman received a very different impression. The following words are hers: "He just was mad at me for telling him his business, so he punished me by not treating my child. He wouldn't give me any medicine. They were all like that. They came and went (from our clinics) and didn't really care. And when they did do something, it was just to give pills out. And this time,

when I needed pills for my baby, he wouldn't give them to me. He was a big shot there so who could I argue with? I went back three times, questioning him—I know it was disrespectful, but I had to. Besides, he thought I was just an Indian who wasn't as smart as him. I went home that night, like I did the whole week, without any help.

"I held Stacy close to me in the bed as she slept. I didn't want to sleep, because I kept hearing her breathe hard, loud, squeaky sounds. I was scared. I held her propped up so she wouldn't drown in her snot. I was so tired and stressed I fell asleep. The next morning, Stacy was cold. The noises were gone. She was dead. And nobody cared. I didn't have my baby no more. I didn't have my womanhood—my family saw to that, tying up my tubes. My baby was dead and there would be no more. Stacy was gone and so were all the others."

I sat there. Quiet, respectful tears streamed down my face. I honored her pain with my tears. After much silence, she said, "I share this story with you because you know the way of harmony and how to teach me to get there. You believed I was in pain and looked for the reasons. The energy healings have eased my pain and helped me speak of this thing I have carried inside." Few providers had taken the time to include her in a participatory relationship. In this caring environment, Patricia's pain, once carried deep within her heart, broke free and she began to be healed. ∎

Rosze Barrington, MS, RN, ANP, CS
1995

JACK

My first encounter with Jack came shortly after I started working in the office of a busy HIV physician's practice. Even though our patients had appointments, they were booked every 15 minutes, usually making the wait 2 hours or more. When I called Jack into the exam room, he handed me a box of chocolates. With a big grin on his face, he said, "This is my secret weapon for winning over the staff and getting in to see the doctor within 2 hours." Jack's face was mischievous. He had disarming blue eyes and an engaging smile that forced you to join him in his conspiracy. No matter how stressful the day was, I could always count on Jack to make me laugh. I looked forward to his office visits.

A year later, when I left the office and moved into homecare as a nursing supervisor, I happened to find Jack under my care again. By now, he had nurses' aides to assist him around the clock with bathing, meals, and general housekeeping chores. Jack didn't need this extensive care, but he knew how to get what he wanted. His profession had been in the movie industry, and his influence was evident by the numerous photographs that surrounded him in every room—his 'family,' as he referred to them. Whenever I visited Jack, he was holding court with his many friends, telling stories and enjoying the attention bestowed upon a dying man.

Jack and I spoke often about his deteriorating health and about what he wanted to do when he was near the end. Although Jack had been a monk in the past and still had a very strong Catholic faith, he decided to die at home and not be admitted to the Catholic hospital when the time came. He would say repeatedly, "I want to be surrounded by the love of my friends," referring to his photographs. Over the years we established a relationship that was deep, although usually illustrated by continual banter. The nature of our relationship allowed us several levels of intimacy that extended beyond the typical patient–nurse relationship.

One night I received a phone call at 4 am. It was Jack's aide, frantically telling me that Jack was dying, and that he was demanding to be taken to a Catholic hospital. After all of our conversations, I could hardly believe what I was hearing. We had discussed this moment several times and worked hard to assure that Jack would stay home.

Frustrated and angry, I arrived at Jack's place as the ambulance arrived. While the attendants were rolling their gurney into his small apartment, I went to check on Jack. Despite his gaunt appearance and slow, purposeful gestures, Jack was barking out orders to his aide,

156

"...and get the two pictures on the table over there, and the smaller one by my bed, and don't forget the yellow cardigan sweater..." It was futile to get Jack to relax and listen to the ambulance attendants. Jack demanded "I want to sit up so I can see where we're going." As we moved his patio flowerpots to make room for the gurney, Jack shouted to the attendant, "Move that pot over there so you don't break it!"

Feeling the frustration and tension, I attempted to interrupt Jack's tirade. I blurted out from behind the gurney, "For God's sake, Jack, would you just lie back and let these men do their job? The next thing you'll be doing is telling the grave diggers how to throw the dirt on your casket!" Immediately Jack stopped giving orders. He lay back and was silent for the entire ride to the hospital. I feared that my attempt to calm the situation had overstepped the bounds of our relationship and damaged Jack's floundering attempts to maintain control.

After he was admitted to the hospital, I promised Jack that I would visit him when I got off work. My stomach turned in anguish all day over how I would apologize to him for what I had said. I did not know what it would take to mend our relationship and, equally important, restore his power to him. I arrived at Jack's hospital room only to find him once more holding court with his friends. As I stood in the doorway, Jack looked up at me with his radiant smile and laughingly said "The next thing you'll be doing is telling the grave diggers how to throw the dirt on your casket." I knew that all was forgiven and that all would be fine as I stepped into the room and joined in the laughter. My risky comment worked without damaging our relationship, and it provided a means to further enhance our mutual respect and trust. ∎

Edward L. Seefried, RN
1989

ANNABELLE

The first time I saw Annabelle she was walking toward our medical team in Zacatecas, Mexico. She leaned on her mother for support because she had a severe limp. Her deformed right leg made it difficult and painful for her to walk. She and her mother had heard about our medical team and came to ask for help.

Annabelle had injured her knee when she was a small child. A plate and screws were put in to help the knee heal. After an infection, the metal was removed, and the deformity developed over the years as she grew into her teens. Team physicians studied x-rays and examined Annabelle and determined she would need a major surgical procedure to straighten her leg and make it easier for her to walk. Surgery of this type is complex by American standards. This was something that the team could not do in Mexico.

Our team was in its early years and we had not yet brought a patient from so far away to the States for surgery. All the logistics would have to be worked out—it seemed as though it would be almost impossible. Annabelle said she would keep hope and pray that we would help her and would someday send for her. As we said our good-byes she reached up and unfastened the chain from her neck. On the chain was a little medal, which her mother said she wore all the time. She reached up and put the medal and chain around my neck and said "This will help you remember me, keep it until I come to San Diego, then you can give it back ."

Time went by and the international logistics were worked out. Annabelle came to San Diego and had her surgery. The procedure lasted for more than 8 hours, followed by several weeks of physical therapy and a special brace to help with walking. Soon she was able to return home. As she was leaving, I slipped the chain from my neck to give back the medal and she stopped me and said "Please keep it, and remember there are other children who need your help."

I have never forgotten. Since that time, our team has helped more than 2000 children have a chance for a better life through corrective surgery for cleft lips, cleft palates, burn scars, hernias, orthopedic problems, and other conditions.

I often think of Annabelle—how impossible it all seemed and how the faith of one young lady helped us help her. This faith gives us the inspiration to continue our work. ∎

Patricia Robinson, BSN, RN

MRS. BENITO AND FAMILY

I am a post anesthesia care unit (PACU) nurse and most of my contact with the patient ends when they leave this unit. On one particular occasion, I had to accompany our orderly to transport a patient in a large bed to her hospital room. Mrs. Benito was an elderly, slightly confused woman who had recovered well from a total hip replacement surgery.

We stopped outside the waiting room as is our policy, to see if any family was there. Upon announcing her name, a small dapper man presented himself as her husband. Late 80s, suit, wire-rim glasses, and as cute as could be. He warmly greeted Mrs. Benito and accompanied us upstairs. He held her hand, patted her arm, and whispered words of encouragement. She in turn, although pretty sleepy from the pain medicine, told him not to worry, smiled, and squeezed his hand in return.

There was more family in her room who were forced to point out that the elderly man was not her husband, as he had passed away years ago. Luckily, the alleged husband was easily escorted back to the waiting room to his real family, who thought he had gone to the restroom. Yes, he was also somewhat confused and his real wife was still in surgery! ∎

Christine Rodighiero, RN
1995

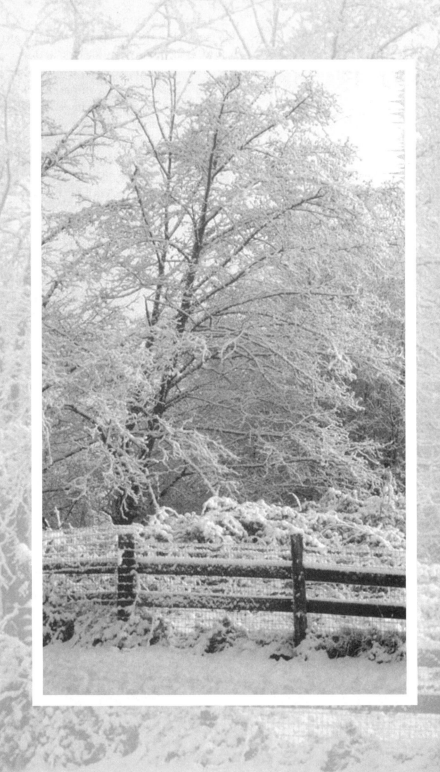

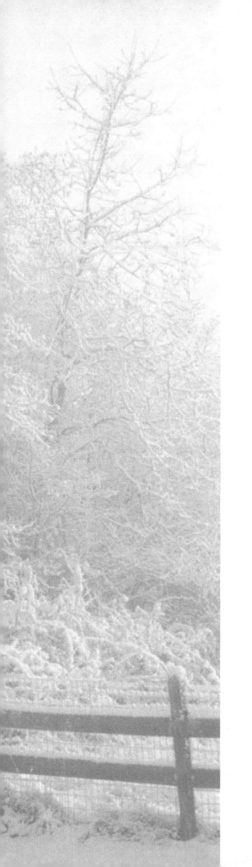

PEACE

JAKE AND REBECCA

Time seemed to drag from the moment I knocked until he opened the front door to the apartment. Dressed in a long-sleeved shirt and tie, Jake offered his right hand to shake with mine as he muttered hello. His eyes and smile beamed at me as he slowly walked, with cane in hand. A woman sat in the living room; he introduced her as his wife, Rebecca. She seemed perfectly capable and I wondered why she hadn't answered the door. I didn't ask and went on to perform the tasks I had to do. I had six patients to see that day, so when Jake asked me if I'd like a cup of tea, I declined.

I visited him for about 4 weeks. I watched him struggle to answer the door, struggle to learn his medications, struggle to learn to take care of himself independently. Yet he was always pleasant, and his wife always stood by watching and encouraging. Jake never complained about his condition and he always complimented the physical therapist and me for helping him to recover. At each visit he offered me a cup of tea.

I always walked away confused about his attitude. Jake would say he was thankful to be alive and didn't seem to notice his disability—other than the fact that it took him so much longer to perform the simple tasks.

One day I stood in front of Jake and Rebecca's door waiting for it to open. Rebecca answered and said Jake was still getting dressed but I could see him in the bedroom. Jake extended his hand as was his customary greeting to me, and my eyes were immediately drawn to a set of numbers etched into his forearm near his wrist. I looked up into his eyes and he smiled. My hand slipped out of his, and I sat down, waiting for him to continue dressing.

Suddenly it all made sense. Rebecca honored his desire to remain independent by simply walking alongside him on his path of recovery. He was happy to be alive, so grateful to have come this far after being a victim of the Holocaust. And every moment was precious, deserving of a bit of conversation and cup of tea.

His vital signs were within normal limits. As I put away my equipment, I heard him say, "Cup of tea, nurse?" I felt honored to be in the presence of someone so humble, with such dignity.

"I take just milk, Jake. Thank you." Rebecca made her way to the kitchen as we convened in the dining room. The fresh flowers on the dining room table smelled heavenly. We laughed our way through some stories and I got up to leave. I thanked them for being a gentle reminder to take time to be grateful for what you have no matter how difficult the circumstances may seem. ∎

Karen Bauer, MS, RN
1984

162

SARAH, JESSICA, ALLISON, AND JOHN

In my role as a psychiatry consultation liaison nurse, I received an urgent page from the intensive care unit. John, a 41-year-old man whom I had never met, had just died, after a relatively brief admission. Allison, his fatigued and grieving wife, wanted to bring their two daughters, ages 5 and 7, in to say good-bye to their dad. She was not sure what to tell her daughters or how to prepare them for what they would see. John's nurse, Chris, was providing postmortem care. Could I help?

Upon arrival in the ICU, Chris provided me with a summary of what had happened. I proceeded to the family room where I met Allison, Sarah, age 7, and Jessica, age 5. With their mom's permission I explained what had happened to their dad, ending with the fact that he had died. As a nurse who works mainly with adults, I carefully chose words and phrases that a 5- and 7-year-old would understand. Their mom held both the girls at her side but, due to her own grief, was not able to say much. When given the opportunity, the girls asked questions like "Why did this happen to my dad?" and "Does he hurt anymore?" Allison and I responded to these questions as best we could.

Since they were from a community several hundred miles from our hospital, I wanted the girls to be able to say good-bye to their dad before they left. I gently asked if they wanted to see Daddy before they went home. Both little ones, with their beautiful big brown eyes, nodded 'yes'. We spent some time talking about what they would see—some of the equipment and the fact that Daddy would look different.

We were ready. Sarah and Jessica took my hands and we walked down what seemed to be a much longer hallway than usual, into the ICU. Chris met us at the entrance to John's cubicle and the five of us entered a quiet little part of the ICU—a part of the ICU covered with little children's pictures and cards. While Chris stayed at Allison's side, I walked slowly to the bedside with Sarah and Jessica. They were quiet and tentative, Sarah gently touching her dad's hand. "Why is he so cold?" "Why is he so white?"

I carefully answered their questions and let them be with their dad. The girls said they were ready to go. I asked if they would like to pick out one of their pictures to send with Daddy. They each solemnly picked out a picture and Chris promised to send them with John.

Just before we left the cubicle, Jessica pulled at my sleeve and pointed to a balloon bouquet tied to John's bed. I knelt down and asked her what she wanted. She replied "I want to take them home and put them out my bedroom window so when Daddy looks down from Heaven, he'll know where Sarah and I are." I untied the balloons. Sarah, Jessica with balloons clutched in her hand, and I walked out of the ICU. By then, the family had arrived and I said a tearful good-bye to Allison, Sarah, and Jessica. Allison quietly mouthed "Thanks" as the elevator doors closed.

I believe I was able to ease the distress of a young woman by providing support and compassion to her children. I was honored to be present at a most personal, intimate moment in a family's life. What a gift our profession gives us. ■

Linda Newton, MN, RN, CPMHN(C)
1996

LYNDA

I practiced in pediatric oncology and trauma before the AIDS epidemic. Death and I know each other very well. Maybe that is why I had been thinking about leaving, getting out of the business.

The rodeo will have to wait. Lynda was the first patient in my primary care nurse practitioner practice when I moved to Cape Cod. The first time we met, she sat across from me in a methadone clinic. Lynda had been brought in by one of her counselors for some infraction of the rules. The counselor was talking about rules that seemed to have nothing to do with staying clean and sober and living with HIV. By the time the counselor finished, the tension in the room was explosive. Lynda calmly stood and announced, "You're an ass."

As Lynda turned to leave, she said to me "So you gonna help me or what?"

"Sure," I replied.

So it began. I helped Lynda get off methadone. She taught me about addicts and addiction. Life was hard for her. Life was also very good because she loved it so. She always dreamed. She believed she would outlive the virus. And, I guess, so did I. Lynda was always there.

Rick Ferri, PhD, RN, ANP, ACRN
1997

She was not easy to get along with. In fact, she could be a major pain. Yet, we connected in a special way. She would yell and I would yell back. She would make outrageous demands and I would meet them. She hated that. This was not a typical nurse–patient relationship.

But Lynda frequently reminded me if I wanted a patient I could go to a hospital.

She was also vulnerable and needed to be accepted. Lynda knew that no matter what happened, we would be OK. Lynda became my patient, friend, and mentor. Lynda would sit on her porch as I ran by her house each morning and she would yell after me. I always stopped on the way back to talk.

I have learned a lot in this epidemic and Lynda was one of my main teachers. She forced me to re-examine how I approached all my patients. She demanded that the barriers of superiority that accompany the health provider professions be brought down. She forced the human agenda.

However, my girlfriend died and I cried. There was a hidden part of my heart that was revealed by my work and relationship with Lynda. I didn't even know I still had it. I cared. I cared a lot.

Two nights before she died, I was sitting in her living room talking to her about her medications. It was just a regular visit, nothing out of the ordinary. Except that I had a great feeling of satisfaction come over me. I could feel the restlessness of my desire to leave AIDS care vanish. I felt at home once again. ∎

165

MAMORU M.

I am the first and the only psychiatric liaison clinical nurse specialist in a 637-bed municipal hospital in a large Japanese city. One day, the nurse of the internal medicine unit asked me to see a patient named Mamoru M. Mamoru M. was 71 years old. He suffered from stomach cancer and pneumonia. Responding to such a request was part of the role I helped to develop at the hospital.

His wife pushed him in a wheelchair as they came into the interview room. He was extremely thin and looked pale. However, when he saw me, he greeted me politely and began to talk quietly. "I am conscious that death approaches. But I am anxious about dying. I don't know how to die in the best way, a good way. I don't know how to part from the important people in my life. I wanted to know the method that would ease this worry, so I asked for the interview." I told him "It is very important work to think about death and dying." His wife nestled close to him and sat quietly. After listening to him, she said "I cannot think of you dying." As he saw his wife shedding tears, he said "I will die soon."

Tearfully, he told the story of how he nursed his mother during her terminal illness. "Until she died, I nursed my mother for 4 months.

My mother suffered badly because of the illness. But, even though her condition was very bad, she died well. She did not forget to say thank you and show her appreciation to the people in the neighborhood to the end. She was always resolute." He began to speak about the way that he had lived. "I am the eldest of six sons, the brother who could be respected as a model all the time. And I was respected by my colleagues at the workplace and people in the neighborhood, too."

He remained silent for awhile after talking of his life. I said "You want to die resolutely in the same way as your mother and as you have been in your life until now. But you are suffering because it can't be done so." He nodded slowly, deeply and said "I am shameful." He then said, "Let me cry here" and cried loudly.

To comfort him, I rubbed his back as he spoke and cried. I told him "You have lived well. You are trying to think about your death and dying firmly. You don't need to ever feel shameful. Your attitude can be respected very much. From now on, let's think about your death and dying together." We planned another visit.

Over the course of the next week, his condition worsened rapidly. I visited his room. His wife, five younger brothers, a doctor, and a nurse were around his bed. He saw me and stretched his hand toward me—a hand that had become even thinner. Then, putting his hands together before his face, he said to me "I have a wish. Make me breathe easier."

The pneumonia had worsened, with a remarkable decline in his pulmonary function. He required an intravenous drip of morphine prescribed by the doctor. Now, breathing more easily was more important than controlling the pain. Using morphine under the present conditions could cause sedation. The doctor told him that it was possibile he would not wake up after morphine was given. Mamoru M. nodded deeply. And he said "please" again.

I wanted to know how he got along with his wife and younger brothers since our first interview. Will he recover his dignity? I thought that not only I, but also all the people in the room had to hear his answer. I asked "Could you tell your younger brothers what you wanted to tell them?" He nodded yes. Then he looked over at his wife and younger brothers. His younger brothers said "We talked very much. We always gathered together and talked as our usual family practice, because our older brother was a good adviser. We have talked fully with our older brother. It is sufficient now. Our older brother did his best. Do as our older brother says, please." His wife nodded, too.

The doctor, the nurse, and I looked at him. He looked at us too. His attitude was calm, though he was having a hard time breathing. I understood that Mamoru M. had recovered his dignity. He was there as an older brother and a husband who could be respected by his younger brothers and his wife. The doctor looked back at me and I nodded. In the beginning, the doctor seemed reluctant to use morphine. After observing my intervention, listening to the family, and seeing my confidence, it seemed the decision was made. The doctor told him, "Let's use morphine."

Mamoru M. and his family looked relieved. I told him "You are allowed to be able to talk with your wife and your younger brothers. It is good when breathing becomes easy." He nodded, took my hand, and said "Thank you." I held his hand and nodded.

He was liberated from the congestion, though the morphine was only a small dose. But his condition worsened and his consciousness declined gradually.

During Mamoru M.'s dying, I allowed him to cry as deeply as he felt. Many Japanese men think it is shameful to express worry and emotion, feel loneliness, and lose the opportunity to reform their heart. Mamoru M.'s heart was healed and he could change the way he interacted with his family.

Mamoru M. was a respectable eldest son for the younger brothers, and he was a respectable husband for his wife to the end. He took himself back, regaining his dignity and self-respect with gentleness and resolution, and died. ∎

Kiyoka Nozue, PhD, RN, PLCNS
1997

IDA

Ida was 82 when we met. I was a nursing student working in a general practitioner's office. My heart was set on becoming a nurse. Though I was not yet a registered nurse, Ida would teach me a nursing lesson that remains with me 24 years later.

One day Dr. Lindsey, my employer and Ida's doctor, asked if I could help provide transportation for her. Unaware of the consequences, I agreed to help.

Ida had multiple health problems, including cellulitis in her legs. I was astonished the first time I visited Ida. She lived in a small building, the size of a one-car garage. It had only a dirt floor. Ida had several layers of wall-paper hung from the ceiling, creating a bedroom/sitting room and kitchen. There was no telephone service and no running water. A neighbor brought a bucket of water each day.

A large radiator in the middle of the bedroom/sitting room kept the temperature at 90° in winter and summer. Ida also used the radiator for cooking.

In my zest to be helpful, I offered to shop for Ida. Her grocery list con-sisted of crackers, cheese spread, shredded chicken lunchmeat, ice cream, and 68 to 78 cans of cat food, depending on how many cats she was caring for at the time. I suggested that Ida keep fewer cats, which would allow more money for the purchase of healthy food for her. Indignantly, Ida explained "Life is full of choices. I choose to take care of cats. My kitties do more for me than food."

One day I delivered groceries and stayed to chat. A pie tin of cat food sat on the folding chair next to mine. While we were talking, two moles waddled out from under Ida's bed, shimmied up the leg of the chair, and plopped down in the pie tin. Noticing my shock, Ida said "I figure that as long as there is enough to go around, it doesn't hurt to share the goods."

Ida and I talked about many things through the years. She explained that when she died she wanted her kitties put to sleep "because no one can take care of my kitties like I can." Ida's 90° home, with its 15 cats, two moles, and the neighbors' chickens and ducks, was a breeding ground for many critters. Frequently, Ida opened her door, allowing the breeze to cool her room, but with the breeze came the local wildlife. On one occasion, a pheasant met me in the kitchen.

I took a special dinner to Ida on the afternoon of her final Christmas. It seemed drafty in her sitting room and I discovered that a cat had fallen through the kitchen roof. There was an inch of snow covering the floor and the dead cat. I asked Ida if she had been out to the kitchen. "No, I've been chilly," she answered, "so I stayed in bed."

I felt so sad telling her about her kitty and the roof, especially on Christmas Day. Ida replied "Well, it's better to die active than just waste away—besides, we will always remember that kitty died on a special day." Ida never named her cats; there were too many.

Her philosophy was simple, yet profound. Ida had three dresses and washed them in a wooden bucket. She dried the dresses by hanging them above the radiator. I suggested that her method for drying the laundry might be a fire hazard. I realized that I wasn't going to change 80 years of living. She would say "I know you mean well, but it just won't work for me."

As a student nurse, I was sensitive to Ida's chiding. Everyone is unique, special unto their own right, with their own set of values and priorities. As a nurse, and a person, I am not there to judge, but to help. Ida's definition of health was a stark contrast to what I was learning in nursing school and was sometimes difficult to accept.

Shortly before Ida died, she gave me a pair of white linen dress gloves. "I want you to have these" she said. "I worked hard to buy these gloves for my high school prom. The boy who asked me never showed up. I've never had an occasion to wear them, but I thought you might be able to use them." "Thank you" I said, somewhat puzzled about the sudden gift. Ida must have sensed my confusion, because she continued. "You have given me something very valuable and I want you to have something special too."

I thought she was thanking me for grocery shopping, for taking her to the doctor, the hospital, the bank, or getting the roof fixed at Christmas. "What did I give you Ida?" I asked. "These gloves are to thank you for giving me dignity, not questioning the way I live, and understanding that I must keep my integrity to live. This has been a very special gift, and I want to thank you." She placed the gloves in my hands.

Ida died 2 months later, in her home, alone. By the time Dr. Lindsey notified me, the city had razed Ida's home. I called the city and learned that they had put all the kitties to sleep.

Since that time, I completed nursing school and have practiced in cardiovascular nursing as a manager, an instructor, researcher, and a health care consultant. Ten years ago I began working in home health care and rekindled the joy of knowing my patients, their families and pets, well. It's curious that I have found success and joy in home health care nursing. However, no patient situation has ever compared with Ida's.

I still have Ida's gloves. I keep them in the top drawer of my dresser. Every now and then I take them out and remember—each of us is an individual with a unique sense of dignity and integrity. This truth, acknowledged without bias, can be the best nursing intervention of all. ∎

Ann K. Frantz, BSN, RN
1970

CARLOS
AND STEVE

Near Christmas time, our AIDS care unit was busier than ever. All of the patients were very sick. One patient, Carlos, was near the end-stages of his life. He had been on the ward for 3 weeks after a week-long admission to the ICU for severe electrolyte imbalance. Carlos had severe diarrhea, which required measuring the amounts every 2 hours. We then replaced the amount with IV solutions. He had multiple IV lines that had a long succession of potassium, magnesium, intravenous nutrition, lipids, and antibiotics infusing. Carlos was barely responsive and had been this way through his whole admission. He frequently had high fevers. He weighed about 100 lbs. The nurses on the unit frequently commented among themselves "Why won't the physicians give up on Carlos?" Despite his fragile condition and near coma, he lived.

In contrast to Carlos, the young man in the next room down the hall was a 28-year-old attorney named Steve. Steve had been admitted a few days earlier with presumptive pneumocystis pneumonia. He had never been HIV tested, but told us that he was gay and he thought he might in fact be HIV positive.

Steve was admitted to the ward from ED in a 3-piece Brooks Brothers suit. He had tried a case in court the day he was admitted. He told us that he had been so short of breath by the end of the court case that he knew something had to be wrong. By the time he arrived on the floor, his temperature was 104°F and his oxygen saturation level was in the 70s. He was placed on a 100% hi-flow oxygen. Steve continued to be severely short of breath—so short of breath, that to remove his oxygen mask for a few minutes to eat or drink took incredible effort and depleted his energy for several hours. After 48 hours of antibiotics, there didn't seem to be any improvement.

Steve's mother had arrived from out-of-town that afternoon to visit him. The day nurse had reported that his Mom, while being very upset about his condition, had been very kind and loving to him.

That night, another nurse called me into his room. She was trying to get him in a more comfortable position. He seemed particularly agitated and anxious. We did our best to get him propped straight up at a 45-degree angle in bed to assist his breathing. He was even more short of breath than before. We checked his oxygen saturation level and it was falling into the low 80s, rapidly. She quickly placed a call to the intern for assistance. By the time the intern got to the room, Steve was gasping for breath. The intern wanted to try to intubate him, but we quickly reminded him that Steve had requested a 'No Code.' The intern then agreed to give him an injection of morphine to ease his breathing. A few more moments passed, and Steve's breathing eased, slowed, and peacefully stopped.

After I was finished helping my colleague with Steve, I realized that I needed to check on my own patients. Walking down the hall, I stopped at the nurse's desk to tell my co-workers that Steve had just died. We all commented on the fact that Steve, who physically and mentally appeared so robust and healthy, had gone before Carlos, who was so thin and had been at the end-stage of life for so long.

I asked one of my co-workers to help me turn Carlos onto his side. When we went in Carlos' room, we found him wide awake, staring out the window. I said "Carlos, we're going to turn you on your other side now," as I had said many times before. I had never received a response or heard Carlos speak a word. He looked up at me and very clearly said "Did you just hear that knocking at the window?" Shocked that he could even speak, I asked what he was talking about. He said "About 5 minutes ago, there was a man at my window, knocking and motioning for me to follow him. Do you know who he was?" I looked at my co-worker in amazement, for we were on the tenth floor. I questioned him further, "What did he look like, Carlos?" He could not describe the man except to say that he kept trying to get Carlos to follow him.

Carlos did follow him several days later. ∎

Jill Kunkel, RN

ANNE

I was working as a psychiatric liaison clinical nurse specialist in a department of medicine when I was called to see Anne. Her attending physician had requested that I talk to Anne because "she was not dealing appropriately with her diagnosis of pancreatic cancer." As I listened to his discussion of Anne's history, I kept thinking to myself, "How does one deal 'appropriately' with being told you have cancer?" I was perplexed by this situation because pancreatic cancer is known to be deadly, and the prognosis is 1 to 2 years of survival after being diagnosed. From Anne's history, she had been having symptoms for at least a year.

I entered Anne's room. I told her that her doctor had wanted me to talk to her because she had been diagnosed with cancer, and he was concerned with how she was dealing with the diagnosis. She looked at me and said "Not well. I mean, is it normal to be thinking about your funeral and how you want things done?" I shook my head and continued to look at her because I did not think that she was finished with what she wanted to say.

"You know, I've done a lot of reading about the pancreas. I've gone to medical school libraries to check out books and read journal articles about the different

pancreatic disorders. You see, I've had these pancreatic symptoms for a year and a half. The doctors haven't been able to find anything definitive until today. This was my third CAT scan and the cancer finally showed up on this scan. So, you see, I know that I don't have much time to live."

As I sat listening to her talk, I kept thinking to myself that this lady knows herself and knows what she wants to do. Now, whether the doctors or her family will allow her to do what she wants is another story. And I also knew that she was correct about not having long to live.

As I nodded my head in agreement, Anne continued to say "How do you tell your husband that you love that you are dying? How do I tell my two daughters that I won't be here much longer? Am I insane to be thinking about my funeral? You know, they [her husband and daughters] won't know where to begin." I looked at Anne and said "No, it's not insane to be thinking about your funeral. Remember, though, you have been reading about the pancreas and its disorders for a long time. You have been worried that you had pancreatic cancer all this time and now have found out. However, your husband and daughters haven't had the same amount of time to deal with this. It will be a shock to them. Let's progress slower with them."

We discussed how she would talk to her husband and daughters that evening, that she would just talk about her diagnosis, and that she did not have long to live. I returned the next day to find her in better spirits, but still worried about her family. Anne said "They don't want to believe that I don't have much time. They keep telling me that everything will be OK. I guess they feel they have to do that for me." We talked about giving her family time to deal with her diagnosis of cancer, and when would be a good time to talk with her husband about funeral arrangements. She decided that while her family was dealing with her diagnosis, she would write down directions for her funeral and what she wanted done.

During the week that she was in the hospital, we talked daily about her and her family's progress. On Friday when she left the hospital, she decided to tell her husband about her funeral arrangements. I found out that Anne died 6 weeks later. I'm glad that she was able to have the time with her family and plan her funeral for them. It was her last gift to her loved ones. ∎

Jane Bryant Neese, PhD, RN, CS
1984

MRS. JOHNSTON

After many years of ICU nursing, I was quite familiar with the unusual sounds that emanate from this unique environment—ranging from the sick, sometimes dying, patients, to the heart-wrenching tears of family, the groans of pain, the clank, clatter, and beep of equipment, and the occasional sweet 'thank you' when someone gets better.

I had arrived on the unit and started to make rounds. As I came closer to Room 611, I heard the most beautiful, angelic singing I have ever heard, sweetly flowing from Mrs. Johnston's room. It was like I was momentarily transported from the ICU to a corner of paradise.

A 78-year-old woman was sitting in bed all 'dolled-up.' Her two daughters were helping comb her hair and had picked out a lovely pink nightgown. All the time they were singing in three-part harmony.

I stood there transfixed by the music. A warm welcome was extended by Julie, one of Mrs. Johnston's daughters. She invited me to come in and join the singing. The words of the hymn were not familiar, but seemed appropriate.

The next 2 days were a real treat hearing them sing together again. I learned they sang years ago when they were all members of the same church choir.

On day three, Mrs. Johnston's heart and kidney functions—which had only been marginal—went from bad to worse. We worked diligently to get her stabilized, but she was failing fast. I knew she was feeling worse as each hour passed, but she touched my hand and said "I appreciate all you're doing for me, but it's in God's hands."

Previous arrangements had been made with instructions that she was to be a 'no code' in the event of a cardiac or respiratory arrest. As the day hung heavy, I knew it was just a matter of time before Mrs. Johnston's heart would totally fail.

Time came for me to give report to the oncoming nurse. As I stood in the doorway finishing my report, I turned to leave when I heard Mrs. Johnston softly call me back. She said "You can't leave yet without giving me a hug good-bye." I leaned over and Mrs. Johnston kissed my cheek and we hugged each other one last time. I looked back as I left the room. Her eyes were closed now and a smile was on her face.

As I started down the corridor, I heard the slow erratic beeping of her monitor go silent. My tears were flowing as I saw her daughters arrive and walk toward me. They looked at me and knew their beloved mother was gone. They embraced me with a hug and said "We appreciate all you've done for Mom. She's in God's hands now." ∎

Cindy Hess, RN, CNOR
1988

MRS. DOE

While on an advanced nursing rotation in my senior year of a baccalaureate-nursing program, I assumed a 'charge nurse' role on a medical/surgical unit. One evening, I was in charge of three other student nurses.

It was about 9:30 in the evening when a family member of a patient who was not assigned to any of us came running toward the nursing station. I was the only one there and they looked to me for help. The family member said "Please come quickly." Since I couldn't imagine what was awaiting me, I looked down the hallway for help. As I walked toward the room, I could feel a sense of impending doom. I considered "What if someone has just died—will I know what to do?"

As I continued to follow the family member, I saw my clinical instructor in my side vision and motioned her to please follow me. Sure enough, when I entered the room I found that the patient was taking her last breath, and various family members stood by her bed quietly crying.

I walked to the foot of the bed as my instructor walked to the side of the bed. She looked down, lovingly

Luc R. Pelletier, MSN, RN, CS, CPHQ
1978

stroked the woman's forehead and hair, then looked up and asked "How long had your mother been ill?" This started a brief conversation about a long illness. Although there was indeed sadness in the room, you could also feel some quiet relief. I continued to observe my instructor from the foot of the bed. I had never been in the presence of a death, but I was experiencing a reverence that had only been mentioned in my textbooks.

My clinical instructor then asked if the family wanted to stay with their mother a little longer. They said "Yes" and my instructor said, "Luc and I will just fix the bed a bit." Upon saying this, the instructor pulled the nasal cannula off of the woman's face, and we straightened her pillow and her sheets. The instructor placed the woman's hands one on top of the other.

We left the 'Mrs. Doe' with her family and checked in on them frequently. I was shocked and surprised by what I had seen. My instructor took me aside and asked about how I was feeling. I told her that her actions and her loving touch were things that I would remember the rest of my nursing life. And I always have. Her caring, soothing words, and the manner in which she communicated to the grieving family powerfully influenced me. She didn't have to rationalize, explain, or otherwise objectify her actions—I knew exactly what she was 'saying' to the family and was sure that they understood her message, as well. ∎

THE SWANSONS

I was working as the evening supervisor in a small hospital in northern Washington state. Part of my responsibilities included relieving other nurses for their dinner break when we were short-staffed. I received a quick report from the nurse leaving and settled in for 30 minutes.

Tonight, when the floor nurse left for a break, she mentioned in her short report that Mr. Swanson, in Room 326, was dying of lung cancer. He was a 'no code.' I don't know why, but this caught my ear. Mr. Swanson had had terminal cancer for some time; I was told his daughter, son-in-law, and granddaughter were visiting him now. As soon as she left for her break, I wandered down to Room 326.

As I entered the room, I could hear the television and saw a man and woman sitting in chairs watching TV. Leaning on the bedside stand was a younger woman in her late teens or early twenties. . .also watching TV. In the bed was a tiny old man. He was severely thin, very pale, and had an oxygen line running to his nose. What disturbed me was his activity. He wasn't speaking or even moaning, but his hands were flailing wildly in the air, and he was rocking back and forth a little on his pillow. No one was noticing.

I have no idea where my action and words came from—it was automatic and instant. I reached over, turned off the TV, and said "You need to pay attention to your father—he's dying!" His daughter was rightfully shocked. Her finger went up to her lips and she said "SHHH!" I replied, "He knows he's dying and needs to know that he's not alone. Talk to him, tell him you're here." The granddaughter heard what I said and sat down beside her grandfather. She began to talk to him, letting him know that he was not alone, that they were with him, and that they loved him.

Mr. Swanson stopped fighting the air; he settled back on his pillow, with his granddaughter holding his hand and talking to him. In 5 minutes, he stopped breathing. He looked relaxed, as if he were sleeping. His granddaughter cried. His daughter wanted to use the phone to notify other relatives. With her husband by her side, she began making necessary arrangements.

As a critical care nurse and an emergency room nurse, I have witnessed many deaths. I believe this is one of the blessings of being a nurse. I have seen the full circle of life. Both birth and death remind me of the importance of each day, of each moment in my own life, and in the lives of those I love. I am grateful to my patients who taught me this lesson—and to Mr. Swanson, who communicated so clearly during his last moments. ∎

Pat Harris-Murray, MN, RN

KAY

The time had come. During my sister Kay's struggle with breast cancer, I had alternated in the roles of confidante, nurse caregiver, friend, and loving sister. Often the separation of roles became blurred as I attempted to use everything within my power to help her through the progressive stages of her illness. The choices I made at times were difficult, often agonizing. Frequently, they were made with the heart instead of with the knowledge I had gained as a nurse. At times they required all the skill and expertise I had to offer, and yet it didn't seem to be enough. Always, there was a painful awareness of the fragile balance between life and death.

My sister was relatively young when cancer tapped her on the shoulder. She had married and was raising three young teenagers at the time of her mastectomy and subsequent treatment. When the cancer recurred, we shared many hours talking of her life, her children, her dreams. She wanted nothing more than to remain a vital part of our lives and yet, as her illness progressed, we sometimes talked of death.

In one such discussion, she asked me to promise to tell her when her time of death was approaching. She thought that, as a nurse, I might know more or recognize more

clearly than she, what was happening. She wanted to prepare herself, her husband, and especially her children, she said. In my naiveté, I agreed.

What was to be the last hospitalization came all too soon. It became apparent to the medical staff that her body systems were failing one by one as the cancer spread. They communicated the information to me and I realized that the time had come to fulfill my promise. As I agonized over how best to tell her, I recognized that I also had to accept the reality of her loss. There could be no going back for either of us.

And so it was that in the privacy and darkness of her room, in the middle of the night, in the presence of God, and with the illumination of the stars in the night outside, I shared with my sister the news of her leaving this earth soon to enter another Kingdom. I told her it was time now for her to prepare for the future, and to let go of the present. I would help her in any way I could. As we cried together, she reached over to pat my head, and said "I love you."

Early the next morning, as soon as she opened her eyes, she asked to see her children. The next few days passed in a blur as family and friends came to spend a few precious moments with her. Day by day she withdrew more to concentrate on the task ahead. My younger sister and I stayed with her constantly, and over and over again we were struck by her courage, her quiet faith, her love and concern for others, and her trust of us to keep her comfortable and safe until it was time for her to leave us. I was so thankful that as a nurse I knew how to help her. On the afternoon of the fifth day, she stated, "I hope God is ready for me. Finally, I'm ready." And she died.

Over the years since Kay's death, I have relived the promise I gave, the words I shared with her, and the pain and joy of those last moments with her. I have no regrets. In that special glimmer of time with her, my soul was touched, and I shall remain forever changed. ∎

Sandy Gunderson
Goldsmith, MSN, RN, CS
1982

THE
ANDERSON
FAMILY

Early one morning, I approached the door of the medical intensive care unit to begin my shift as a staff nurse. As I passed the family waiting area, I noticed a small group of people clustered together. I immediately recognized the Anderson family. Steven Anderson was a 60-year-old patient who frequently visited our unit in acute respiratory distress. The usual scenario was that he had begun smoking again and his severely damaged lungs just could not handle the stress smoking put on them. We knew his wife and adult children well because they always stayed with him while he was in the intensive care unit. They knew that he should not smoke and felt helpless and unable to help him stop. We also knew they were grateful when we were able to pull off one more miracle.

As I passed through the double doors of the unit to enter the nurse's lounge to take report, I could see that a code was just ending. The emergency team of physicians and nurses had tried to resuscitate a patient whose heart had stopped beating. I didn't know if their efforts had been successful or not, and I wondered if Mr.

Anderson had gone into respiratory arrest.

During report, I learned that Mr. Anderson had died despite heroic efforts on the part of the code team. The nurse going off-duty told me it would be my job to 'finish' the code by gathering his personal belongings for the family, preparing the body for the morgue, disposing of any used equipment, and restocking the emergency cart. When I asked about the family, I was told that they were about to be informed of his death and would visit the body when I was ready.

Although I had been a registered nurse for only 6 months, this wasn't the first time I had helped with these responsibilities—but it was the first time that a patient I knew well had died. The room looked like a war zone. There was used equipment all over the place. The bed and floor were splotchy with blood from various tests. Mr. Anderson's body was askew in the middle of the bed, looking gray and messy. When a nursing assistant joined me, I said, "The family can't see this." He agreed, "We better get going."

Quickly, we gathered several large trash bags and threw away the used supplies. We moved out the IV poles and all the other equipment that was used in the code. We swabbed at the floor to get up the blood smears. Together we changed the sheets. We washed Mr. Anderson's arms and neck to be sure there were no bloody stains. We then put a clean gown on him and stood back to survey the results. While the room and bed certainly looked presentable, Mr. Anderson looked uneasy in death. His thin hair was plastered around his face with sweat from the strain of trying to breathe. He hadn't shaved in several days and his beard was scruffy.

Looking at Mr. Anderson, I commented aloud "I have to do something to help him look more comfortable. I think I'll wash his hair and shave him." For a moment, the assistant looked surprised, so I said "I know we don't usually do this— but I could really use your help." His immediate reply was "Okay."

In just a few minutes, we were able to bathe Mr. Anderson and wash his face and hair. The nursing assistant carefully shaved him. We combed his hair back the way we knew he wore it and placed him in a sleeping position. This time, when we stepped back, I knew we had done our best. I left the room to get his family so they could view the body.

They were weeping quietly in the waiting room. Mrs. Anderson broke down in sobs when she saw me. I took her by the arm and led her and her children into his room. As we walked along the hall, she told me that he had been very sick for several days. "He has had such a hard time."

When she reluctantly entered the room, his wife looked over at her husband's body and stood still. She turned to me and said in a wondering tone, "He looks so peaceful. I can't believe it. Thank God he's at peace." She and her children approached the bedside and said their good-byes gently stroking his head and arms.

I left the unit that day with a new appreciation for the privilege of my role as a nurse in the critical life events of my patients. While I have learned to manage many more complex procedures in my career, I have never forgotten how the very simple act of caring for Mr. Anderson's body provided comfort for his family. ∎

Susan H. Harris, DNSc, RN
1972

GLADYS

I was the evening charge nurse of a 40-bed locked psychiatric unit at the state hospital in Texas for chronically mentally ill adults. Most of these patients had been institutionalized since childhood. I decided to create my own 'music therapy' for the patients and staff. I brought my guitar to the unit, hoping I could spark a sing-a-long on the patio. I also dreamed of finding some small way to break through the mental chains of schiz-ophrenia and psychotic disorders to communicate with my patients on a different level.

I drew a little crowd of curious patients as I toted the guitar out to a picnic table and began to strum. I tried to play old familiar songs that almost everyone would know such as 'You are my Sunshine' and 'Down in the Valley.' The patients seemed to enjoy the music. A few others tried to sing despite being off-key or not remembering the words.

Then there was Gladys. Gladys was a very large woman. She was very disturbed and often had mood swings in which she became violent and difficult to manage. Gladys kept to herself most of the time. She rarely responded when you said hello. But I noticed that when the music began, she would be among the first to arrive. A big smile would grow across her face—the smile was quite noticeable, since Gladys had no teeth. She sang loudly, almost at the top of her lungs. For brief moments, I saw a sparkle in her eye and a sense of appreciation for the music. With this subtle success, I tried to teach the little Shaker Song. Week after week, I included this little song in my sing-a-longs. It was difficult to know if anyone listened or even cared about the words.

One day, I asked the patients for song suggestions. Gladys broke her usual silence and said, "Play the one about the light, the light." "Oh, you mean 'This Little Light of Mine?'" I responded. "No, no, the one about the light, the light" she repeated. I couldn't figure out what Gladys was saying. She was so enthusiastic and emphatic. I didn't want to disappoint her, especially since she so rarely asked for anything or even engaged in conversation.

In desperation, I finally decided to play something, so I started off with the Shaker Song. With great glee, Gladys came up to me and said "That's it! That's it!" It then occurred to me that what she had been saying was the last line of the song, "And when we find ourselves in the place just right, we will be in the valley of love and *DE-LIGHT*!" Gladys had understood more than I would ever know. ∎

Jill Bormann, PhD, RN, CS
1983

MR. COHEN

I was working in a San Francisco community hospital as the nurse manager of a 23-bed skilled nursing unit.

Mr. Cohen was an 89-year-old gentle soul, an extraordinary person. His demeanor was charming and he dignified his illness by graciously accepting the expected outcome, although rightfully struggling with the debilitating effects. Mr. Cohen was diagnosed in the latter stages of lung cancer, which had already metastasized to his bone. It was the aftermath of the 1989 Bay Area earthquake. Everyone's nerves were on edge.

Mr. Cohen was a native San Franciscan and was a youngster during the 1906 earthquake. He felt like an 'old pro' during the 1989 event, and provided comfort to his roommate, fellow residents, and staff who had not experienced an earthquake of this magnitude.

I began to spend time with Mr. Cohen and his family, as his time grew near. Mrs. Cohen visited each evening when her daughter was able to drive her to the hospital. They were loving and attentive to him as both husband and father. He feared that he would pass away without them being present. Mr.

Cohen had confided in his family that he was afraid of dying alone. He wished to have a family member or friend present when his "time had come." Jewish tradition holds dearly the belief that one's passing should be treated with the utmost of dignity and respect. From the moment of death, the body is not to be left alone until after burial.

I was asked by Mr. Cohen to become part of this most intimate and personal experience. I reassured him that other nursing staff members and I would be with him in the absence of his family. I too, realized that I did not wish to die alone, feeling disregarded and unprotected during life's greatest transition.

This was a time of introspection. I began to speak to the issue of death at unit staff meetings. This led to an insightful and emotional value clarification process, which was much needed during this trying time. Mr. Cohen passed away 1 month after the earthquake. He was never alone. We bathed him in a communal and loving way and prepared him to be received by his family later that afternoon. I raised the side rails on his bed for his 'protection' and sat quietly at his side holding his hand.

There was a calming presence that we all acknowledged and appreciated. In preparation for Mr. Cohen's passing and during the actual event, each one of us recognized the gift we had received from this remarkable man, who offered us an example of life's grace and dignity. ∎

Roberta L. Block, MS, RN, CS
1989

182

DOROTHY

The year was 1961, and I was halfway through a 12-month training program to become a certified midwife in Scotland.

It is 2:00 am and the phone is ringing insistently. As the student midwife on call, I awaken and rush to answer. The anxious husband is telling me it is time, and I carefully write the address where the expectant mother lives. I call a taxi and gather all the equipment necessary for the home delivery that the would-be parents have been preparing for. On arrival at the house, Mom is in full labor. It is her second child and she is conducting herself in a calmer state of mind than I am. As a student midwife, I will deliver the baby under the supervision of the district midwife, Dorothy, whom I had already called.

I prepare for the delivery, which is imminent, anxiously asking the husband "Is Dorothy here yet?" His response is negative and he asks me how he can help. I ask him to boil more water, knowing that he is not allowed in the room while his baby is being born. Mom is pushing, and the head is crowning, and the birth is uneventful. I breathe a sigh of relief at the sight of a healthy baby girl crying lustily.

As I care for the baby, Mom calmly informs me that she is having strong contractions; I calmly reply by saying that it is the afterbirth coming. This very stoic lady looks me straight in the eye, and assures me that she is giving birth to another baby. Undiagnosed twins flash into my mind as I look in horror and can see a bulging perineum. My horror turns to terror as I examine my patient and see a pending breech delivery. I have witnessed, but have never performed, a breech delivery. I am totally focused on this delivery when I hear a calm voice behind me saying that I am doing fine. Following Dorothy's instructions, a second baby girl is delivered.

There have been many times in my nursing career that I have reflected back to this incident. And many other incidents occurred during that intense year of training that I am thankful to have completed. It taught me in the areas of professionalism, communication skills, critical thinking, decision making, patient advocacy, and good listening. All these attributes are necessary for a competent, caring nurse. ∎

Carol Bartolotti, RN, C, MPA
1962

RANDY

It was a small community hospital in a mid-sized town, the trauma-receiving hospital for a major part of the county. I was working the 7 pm to 7 am shift in the ICU, assigned to care for a young man with a closed head injury. Randy had been riding his motorcycle without a helmet. He lost control of the bike and hit a tree. He looked almost perfect, no fractures, minimal bruising, muscular, tan, 19 years old.

But his pupils were dilated and did not react to light. He was attached to a ventilator that was breathing for him. He had a catheter in his head measuring the pressure in his brain, intravenous lines provided fluid and medicines, and a tube drained urine from his bladder. "What a tragedy!" everyone said. "What a tragedy," I echoed.

I cared for Randy, measuring his vital signs and neurological responses, assessing his body systems, performing all of those supporting activities to keep his body functioning as well as possible. We waited. Would he wake up? Would he be aware? I talked to him constantly, describing each activity before performing it. Because there was so much equipment surrounding the bed, frequently I would rub his feet to provide some human touch along with the technology. I talked about the weather and described what was happening in the world outside the hospital's walls. And it seemed, although Randy never spoke or moved, that he was aware. I felt someone there, someone listening.

A few days passed, and Randy showed no signs of waking up. He developed a slight case of pneumonia that was treated with antibiotics. His parents arrived from out-of-state. The doctors described the grim situation and minimal chance for survival. Randy's parents were not ready to give up. They brought in family pictures, a poster of his favorite movie star, a tape player, and his favorite tapes. We all spent time with them. We watched and waited. They would visit during the daytime and evening, but the long silent nights belonged to Randy and me.

In the intensive care unit, we check vital signs at least every 2 hours. One night, I had checked them at 2 o'clock. They were stable. Why, why didn't he start to wake up? It had been over a week. The swelling in his brain should be gone by now. The pressure was normal. But his pupils still did not react to light; he did not respond. And yet, as I talked about his care or the weather outside, it seemed that Randy was listening.

It was a wild night in the unit. We admitted two patients and managed a major crisis with another. When I went back into Room 1 at 4 o'clock, something had changed. There was a body in the bed. It breathed. The blood pressure had not changed, the heart rate was stable, but there was no one in the room. The person, the presence who had been there, was gone. I touched him—Randy felt different. Within hours, there were signs that Randy's condition was beginning to deteriorate.

The neurologist spoke to Randy's parents about the tragic turn of events and about organ donation. With assurance that Randy could not recover, his parents decided in favor of donation. In those days, transplant was new. One of the few hospitals in the country performing heart transplants was within 100 miles of us. Preservation techniques were not advanced enough to remove the organs and transport them to the receiving hospital. The entire donor was transferred to the medical center. Then the organs were removed in one operating room while the recipient was prepared nearby.

The team arrived in the early evening to take Randy to the Transplant Center. I assisted the transplant surgeon who had come to prepare Randy for transport. The surgeon was young, the senior resident in the program. "Hello, I'm David," he said and we talked, as doctors and nurses do about the patient. I described the change I had sensed in Randy, how he had been in his body at one point in time, and gone a few hours later. David listened as his hands worked skillfully to change equipment. "I know what you mean," he said, "It almost seems you can sense the spirit leaving the body when that time comes."

I walked with Randy, David, and the rest of the team to the transporting ambulance. As they loaded the stretcher, I squeezed his foot one last time and said good-bye. "What a tragedy," I thought.

It was another long night in the ICU. Room 1 stayed empty, silent, the mattress stripped of linen, Randy's poster still on the wall, family pictures on the night stand, waiting for housekeeping to pack everything away.

The next night when I arrived, there was a message from David for all of us. Randy's heart, kidneys, and corneas had been removed. The heart and kidneys had already been transplanted into waiting patients. Although the recipients were anonymous, he gave a few details that helped us appreciate the importance of the gift. There was another teenager with a new heart, a young father with one of the kidneys, and a teacher with the other. Randy's spirit goes on. ∎

Donna Nolten, MN, RN, C, CNA

EUSTACIA
AND FRANK

Her name was Eustacia and her husband was Frank. They had been married 66 years and adored one another. An immigrant Italian couple, Eustacia was a short, chubby woman; Frank, a tall, wiry man. She called him Papa. Together, they had many children, grandchildren, friends. . .and love.

Eustacia would care for Papa, even though she was a patient along with him in the long-term care facility I worked in as a practical nurse. She had multiple health problems and he had end-stage Alzheimer's. It wasn't called Alzheimer's in those days. . .Papa was 'senile' or, as Eustacia would say 'not right in the head.'

She would bathe him, feed him, sleep next to him, and even chastise him in Italian when he was acting combative and stubborn.

Frank died suddenly one day and it was my duty to tell his loving wife. Her grief was immeasurable.

I spent quite some time sitting with her the day Papa died. I listened to stories of her 'man,' of their children, their home, their life in Italy, then here in the United States. We discovered she and Frank were, in fact, friends with my own grandparents long ago, and it was a treasure for me to hear stories of my own family that day.

I remember, in the midst of her grief, her telling me I had no idea how she was really feeling. She had never felt like this in her life and hoped I never had to in my life. I held her in my arms and listened and cried with her.

Eighteen years later, I held the hand of my dying husband. I heard Eustacia's words again and, somehow, I didn't feel as alone. When he was gone and my friend was holding me, I knew she was right. I really could not have known how it would feel until that moment. I felt her, at that moment though, holding me and easing me through my grief as I had for her years before. ∎

Annetta Parente, LPN
1973

UNCLE NORMAN

Operating room nursing is one of the nursing specialties in which the patient never has an opportunity to develop a rapport with their nurse. When OR nurses greet their patients, they are often already sedated.

Sedated or not, an individual approaching surgery is extremely nervous, anxious, and usually afraid. Surgical nurses quietly go about our duties of protecting the patient's rights, ensuring a safe environment, and participating in the performance of surgery in an attempt to return this individual to a better quality of life.

I have been a surgical nurse for 28 years. In 1981, I was working for a group of surgeons in southern New Jersey. Every day we performed surgery at two different hospitals and made hospital rounds on their patients. My Uncle Norman was being admitted to one of the hospitals because he was experiencing some neurologic symptoms. After a thorough workup, a mass was identified in his brain. This was thought to be a brain abscess. My uncle was scheduled for a brain biopsy. The final diagnosis following the biopsy was glioblastoma, a highly malignant brain tumor.

Christine M. Reed, RN, CNOR
1981

Every day I visited my uncle and encouraged him as he recovered from his recent brain surgery. One particular day I said to him, "Uncle Norman, when you get better, I'll come to your house and we can have a beer together." My uncle was born in Ireland and beer is simply part of life. Much to my surprise, my uncle looked at me and said, "No more beer!"

Plans for my uncle's treatment included radiation therapy. This would require his transfer to another hospital (also one that I went to daily). Uncle Norman did not want to go to the other hospital and really didn't want further treatment. He shared these feelings with me, but went along with the program for the family's sake. The day finally arrived when he was transferred for his cancer treatment.

Aside from being an operating room nurse, I was also a competitive body builder and had recently won the East Coast Championship, landing me on the cover of Atlantic City Magazine. The afternoon of his transfer, I went to visit Uncle Norman. I walked into the room and found the bed empty. Assuming he was having a treatment, I went out to the nurse station to see when he would return. The nurse informed me that he had passed away about an hour ago. I returned to his room. On the bedside table next to the empty bed was a copy of Atlantic City Magazine with my picture. I smiled, turned, and left. I knew that, in some way, I was with Uncle Norman before his death. ∎

CHARLIE

Charlie was my first patient. I became his primary nurse when he was transferred from the ICU after a near fatal suicide attempt. Charlie met all the criteria for a person at high risk for committing suicide. He was an elderly man who had recently lost his wife of 46 years. After her death he began to drink heavily. He began to withdraw from his friends. Charlie was a 'character' in his close-knit Irish neighborhood. He was a retired longshoreman who was feisty, funny, and loved by everyone. His absence one day was quickly noted. Friends broke into his apartment and found him unconscious after a failed overdose and hanging attempt.

Needless to say, Charlie did not take kindly to his new status as a psychiatric patient. He spent hours alone in his room and wouldn't participate in any treatment activities. He was cordial but dismissive of staff attempts to get him to leave his room. In my naiveté, I pursued my new role and duties as his primary nurse with a vengeance. I followed all of the rules of developing the nurse–patient relationship.

Charlie recognized my 'green' status and didn't want me 'to look bad' as he later told me. He started to talk to me about the sense of anger and abandonment he felt since his wife's death. She thought that she was protecting him when she did not tell him about her advanced colon cancer.

As Charlie responded to his antidepressants, he began to pursue his recovery with his usual style. He became the star of the unit. His good cheer and energy inspired other patients to get involved. He 'adopted' a Vietnam veteran who was not responding to medication. He was able to convince him to have shock treatments.

Charlie had little use for psychotherapy. He would get better by doing rather than talking. When he was able to talk about his wife, he became tearful but quickly dismissed his grief. Charlie's treatment involved becoming a hospital volunteer. He once again gained star status. As a member of the transport team, he could out-run men half his age. He worked 7 days a week. He arrived promptly at 8 am.

The seasoned doctors and nurses were wary of his miracle recovery. He would always remain at high risk because of his age, sex, substance abuse, and unresolved loss. He was assigned to an experienced male psychiatrist because of his high-risk status. Charlie, however, could not talk with a man about what he viewed as his weakness. He would come and 'touch base' with me on a regular basis. The decision was made that the physician would follow Charlie, but that it would be less threatening to him if I was the provider of his emotional and social support. I would receive clinical supervision from my nursing director and the physician to help me manage a patient like Charlie.

Charlie dropped by the unit regularly. He would bring me his Social Security and Medicare forms to fill out. He told me his glasses weren't 'good for reading.' I realized Charlie was illiterate. I helped Charlie in other ways. He developed throat cancer and required radiation. I became the person who talked to his oncologist and 'interpreted.' I met frequently with the psychiatrist, who continued to warn me about his high-risk status.

One Sunday Charlie showed up on the unit with doughnuts and newspapers. He entertained all of us with his stories. This was not unusual, however. The next morning I received a call from the Director of Volunteers. Charlie was a half-hour late. We called his friends and they found Charlie. He had hung himself.

My personal grief was intense. I felt I had failed professionally because I had not seen signs of impending suicide. I felt angry.

Many years have passed since this experience. Charlie gave me my first opportunity to be a nurse. I also lost my innocence as a nurse. Despite tremendous efforts to save a patient—no matter what our nursing specialty—we will lose certain patients. I'm not mad at Charlie anymore. ∎

Patricia Reddish, MSN, RN, CS
1975

MISS
GEORGIA

Miss Georgia was from West Virginia when she married and moved to Baltimore with her husband. When I met her, she was more than 70 years old and had lived all her adult life in the city, but she still had the delightful speech pattern of the mountain girl she was in her youth.

She had a difficult life and suffered physical abuse from her alcoholic husband. She had three sons and had lost a daughter, who died at the age of 7. One of Miss Georgia's sons was schizophrenic, and a second son, to whom she was closest and depended upon, died of complications of alcoholism at about age 38. Her third son was very busy working and raising a family. After her husband died, Miss Georgia had episodes of depression and multiple physical health problems.

When I met Miss Georgia, she was recovering from coronary artery bypass surgery, and was depressed and experiencing auditory and visual hallucinations. With the help of a geriatric psychiatrist, I convinced the staff that Miss Georgia would benefit from staying in the nursing home while we adjusted her medications.

Over the years that Miss Georgia lived in the nursing home, she developed trust in the nursing assistants, nurses, and physicians. She had always shouldered the burdens of family life, but she got little love and caring in return. During her first year with us, she was able to grieve for her 38-year-old son, who had died just before her admission to the nursing home. She was hugged a lot and was given special little gifts and treats at this time and at other crisis points.

Throughout the 7 years I knew her, Miss Georgia had many health challenges and several episodes of recurrent depression. However, it was never necessary to admit her to a psychiatric facility. We always managed to help her through these periods and to keep her in the place and with the people who represented safety and stability.

Miss Georgia was my friend and we loved each other. She even participated in the filming of a video designed to help nursing home staff care for elderly residents with depression. She said in that video that being lonely was "the terribl'st feeling in the world," but she added with a beautiful smile that the staff of the nursing home made her laugh.

She enriched my life, and I like to think I touched hers gently, and with healing. We both shed tears as we said good-bye when my career took me to another state. ∎

Karen Stanley, MS, RN, CS
1993

TED

It was the mid-80s. One patient in our ICU was a man in his mid-30s, slowly dying of AIDS. Staff were instructed to be extremely careful when handling any body fluid and, especially, with any sharp instruments or needles. Most of the staff wore gown, gloves, mask, and protective glasses when going into the room for any reason. They spent as little time with Ted as possible.

I was the critical care educator. I went into the room one afternoon to restart Ted's IV. It was a difficult one because most of his veins had already been used, but we managed to find a new site. Because of the possibility of blood being spilled, I wore mask, gloves, and gown. Ted and I talked during the time we were together about how alone he felt. His family no longer communicated with him, his lover had died, and none of his friends visited the hospital. He talked about how the staff avoided spending time in his room and how isolated the protective clothing they wore made him feel. He also understood why they wore it, and said that he probably would too.

We talked to the staff about Ted's feelings and they began to spend more time with him. I visited Ted every day. I tried to wear appropriate protective clothing, depending on the reason for my visit. If it was for a few minutes, just to sit at the bedside and talk, I wore regular clothes.

One day, I reached out and touched his hand while we talked. Ted began to cry. "It has been so long," he said, "since someone touched me unless they absolutely had to." I began to cry too. I held his hand and we talked for a long time. As our visit ended, I leaned over the bed to hug Ted. Concerned for me, he asked if I was sure it was safe. We hugged gently. Holding his hand, I promised to keep visiting. I hope that he felt less alone after the visit.

Ted died that night. I will never forget him. ∎

Donna Nolten, RN, C, MN, CNA
1986

THE HIRSCHS

It had been a relatively quiet morning, which was always a treat for the staff of a busy emergency department. We spent this rare unhurried time chatting and catching up. As the psychiatric clinical nurse specialist, it was my role to provide psychiatric evaluation, referral, and crisis intervention. I was also asked to provide support to family members as they were confronted with tragic news.

I had gone back to my office to attend to some paperwork when one of the nurses came by to tell me that they had just gotten a patient 'in full arrest.' His heart had stopped abruptly and neither the paramedics nor the emergency department team had gotten any response to their resuscitation efforts.

She went on to tell me what she knew about this man. While teaching this morning he had suffered a heart attack right there in the classroom. "He's 87!" she added with amazement. She went on to tell me that he was apparently a very respected teacher who had been at this school for many decades. "He was loved by his students. Even some of the other teachers, including the one who

called the paramedics, had been his students," she added. Those who had been with him at the school on his final morning had told all this to the paramedics, then to the emergency department volunteers, nurses, and doctors. He was described as well-known and a very special person in the community. This was a very big loss.

"His wife is on her way. She doesn't know yet that he has died. Can you be with her when she is told?" I was asked. I then began to mentally prepare myself. One of the things I loved about working in Emergency was the unpredictability of it all. Meeting people at such critical moments in their lives was fascinating to me. I hoped this woman would not be too frail and that the doctor would tell her the sad news gently. While awaiting his wife's arrival, other staff members and a volunteer approached me to ensure that I was aware of the situation. This event was rousing much energy.

When Mrs. Hirsch arrived, she was escorted to the small room off the hallway just the other side of the 'See the Nurse First' sign. We called it the 'consultation room.' It had a few stiff, uncomfortable chairs and, as usual, this day it also held a couple of spare wheelchairs folded up along the wall. It was not a warm setting.

I brought a small box of tissues discreetly held down at my side. I greeted Mrs. Hirsch and told her my name. The doctor was there at the same time and we moved into our places. I sat next to Mrs. Hirsch and the doctor sat across from us both. He leaned toward her and told her the story of Mr. Hirsch's death. . .that his heart had stopped and everything was done for him that could be done, but he didn't make it. I was grateful for his manner. His warmth and concern made up for the stark setting.

At that moment I poised myself for her reaction. I had noticed that she was a sturdy and healthy-looking woman, much younger than her 80 years. She had an impressive air of calm about her. I wondered if she was numb. . .I touched the hand on her lap and she softly cried. Without hesitation she announced to us "We were married 59 years—he was my whole life." With that I slipped her a few tissues with which she dabbed her eyes, caught her breath, and said longingly, "I want to see him."

This had been anticipated. Mr. Hirsch's body had been prepared, covered, and moved to the 'isolation room' for privacy. As we stood to take her to him, the doctor expressed his sympathy, reached out and held her hand briefly, and left her with me. We walked in silence toward the room at the farthest corner of the department. She was holding my arm for support as we walked down the hallway. She told me that her husband was a wonderful teacher and that he died doing what he loved. There was comfort in this thought. I put my hand lightly on hers. When we arrived at the room I opened the door solemnly asking, "Would you like some time alone?" Her response was to hold onto my arm tighter. I enveloped her hand with mine as she squeezed my arm. I felt her body lean into mine and I stood firmly to steady her.

We entered the cool room and saw Mr. Hirsch lying on the gurney with a crisp white sheet up to his neck. She let go of my arm and stepped forward. I stayed behind her. Imploringly, she said "Oh, Seymour, I'll miss you so much. I don't know what I'll do without you!" Although surprised by her articulate greeting, I instinctively put my hand gently on her shoulder. A lump rose in my throat. She did not touch him, but stood at the end of the gurney, looking at his face, then moved around to the side.

There was a bond between them. It warmed the room. It struck me that she was connecting with him without touching. (Looking back now I believe she didn't touch him out of respect for their religious custom.) She continued to speak to him as if he could hear her. Softly and tearfully she bid him, "Good-bye . . . I love you . . . Thank you for our 60 years together. . . ." She reached back, took hold of my arm, and drew me to her side. I suppressed a gasp as she continued to pay tribute to him as a wonderful husband, father, and teacher, whose life and work touched many others.

She again leaned on me and let me comfort her with my arm

around her shoulder. My eyes were filled with tears that began to trickle down my cheeks. All was exquisitely serene. Her abundant grace and dignity took my breath away. In spite of her grief, I sensed that she fully accepted his inevitable passage from life. Had she ever imagined this moment, I wondered?

I was completely in awe and choked with tears. I felt a strange mixture of sadness and exultation. I regretted never having known this man. Here I was bearing witness to this woman's spontaneous testimonial upon her husband's death. They had realized an ideal and enduring loving partnership. Her obvious pride in him and their life together moved me intensely.

As we left him I affirmed what I felt and told Mrs. Hirsch, "I wish I had known him." That was the most comforting thing I had to give her. She silently acknowledged my understanding of what she had just shared with me.

I can still see and feel that moment even after all these years. I wanted what they had. I projected myself into the scene before me, imagining some 50-plus years ahead. . .saying my good-byes to a life-long partner. . .with sorrow . . .sweetened by the rapture of fulfilled love and an actualized life. I am forever grateful to the Hirschs for showing me authentic, inspired love, and for the privilege of being their nurse. . .for that moment. ■

Marilyn Shirk, MSN, RN
1982

FLORA

I was a fairly new psychiatric consultation liaison nurse. My role was still a little blurred. I did a little bit of everything.

The nurses asked me to see an elderly woman named Flora to 'tell' her she just couldn't return to the house she'd lived in for years—the house that held her prized piano where she still gave voice lessons, even though she was 90-something. Everyone agreed it was time. But no one wanted to tell Flora. Flora had been a Viennese opera singer. She had survived the Nazi concentration camps by literally singing for her life in Teresenstadt.

So, I went down to the room at the end of the hall to talk with Flora. She was a bird-like little woman, completely blind, with an elegant voice. I sat down in the chair next to the bed and began to hem and haw about the difficulties, the losses associated with aging . . . and the strangest thing happened. Flora stopped me, rescued me, really. She took my hand, and said these words I have never forgotten: "Listen, my dear. I did not live to be nearly 100 years old without making the changes I needed to make, when I needed to make them." Flora went on to tell me she certainly understood that it was time to move to the assisted living apartments.

This was the beginning of a very special relationship for both of us. Flora was in and out of the hospital for various things, and I always visited with her. She told me incredible stories about her life; but, while she had a remarkable memory, she did not live in the past. She would listen to opera, but sang 'Making Whoopie!!' and 'Diamonds Are A Girl's Best Friend' at the talent show where she now lived. Flora lived to be more than 100 years old . . . 100 and something—I'm not sure what.

When she could no longer manage at assisted living, she decided she'd had enough life and came to the hospital to die. We spent some time together before she died. I supported her in her decision to make the 'final change,' and assured her I would attend her memorial service when she voiced concerns no one was left alive to be there.

It was an incredible memorial service, simple and elegant, as she wanted. Her 86-year-old brother gave the eulogy. The Rabbi played the soprano's part—Flora's part—from one of her favorite operas. The light streamed in through the stained glass windows in the tiny chapel, blessing a life well lived, and a death accepted as the final change in life. ∎

Kelly Gaul, MSN, RN, CS
1998

RAY

During the years I functioned as a mental health consultant, staff called me when they encountered problematic or perplexing patients and families. I was surprised when Sarah called me. She exhibited great compassion and ability to communicate effectively.

Ray was a 47-year-old experiencing chest pain, increasingly unabated by medication. A heart catheterization revealed blockage in several arteries. Surgery to correct the blockage was recommended, but since Ray declined surgery, he was scheduled for discharge.

Sarah was clearly perplexed. How could someone as intelligent as Ray elect not to have a treatment intended to improve quality of life? The frustrated physician saw no recourse except to prescribe medication and discharge Ray. Sarah thought I might be able to determine why he refused surgery. Thus far he offered no reasons.

I suggested we talk with Ray together. This would maintain the primary therapeutic relationship between them and allow Sarah to observe my interaction.

Once Sarah obtained Ray's permission, we proceeded. I pointed out that while Sarah's area of expertise was the heart, mine was talking with people. I helped figure out puzzling situations. Ray

agreed to talk but didn't think he could shed much light on the situation. He did not want the surgery.

I started out with a familiar hospital approach. "I know you have probably told many people your medical history, but when did the chest pain begin?"

As he talked, I gently guided him to tell more about himself. Without being intrusive, I helped him talk about his life, work, and family.

As Ray described his family, he began to fidget. I sensed some conflict existed here. Gently, I asked more about these relationships. He said "I feel good about the way my kids have turned out."

"And your relationship with your wife Ray?"

"We're really different."

"How do you mean? You like different things?"

"My wife likes nice things, comfortable things."

"What do you like, Ray?"

"I like simple things."

"If you could do anything you wanted, what would it be?"

He paused, looking out the window. His eyes began to shine. "There's a place up north, in the woods, by a lake." He described a small piece of land in a rugged wilderness area. He sighed, "I'd really like to live there."

"That must be tough for you. It doesn't sound like a place your wife would enjoy."

"Not at all. She doesn't even like to go camping. When the kids were small, I thought it was just too much for her to deal with, but now, it's no different. She had a fit when I suggested it. I'm not surprised. It's just the latest in a lot of things we haven't seen eye to eye on—for years."

While Ray seemed at ease from the outset, I noticed increased animation as he described this special place.

I decided to take a risk. "What makes you stay in the marriage?"

"My wife's family, I guess. They're very much like her—or she's like them, very proper. Divorce is not an option. I wouldn't want to do that to her. I love her. I'm just not 'in love' with her anymore."

"So the only way out is to die."

He started to object, then suddenly stopped. "I hadn't thought of it that way, but . . . that's right. (Another long pause) I'm amazed. I've never talked with anyone about this."

"You really are struggling, aren't you? You don't want your wife to be humiliated. Rather than end a marriage that's not working, you're choosing the only acceptable way out—death."

"I hadn't realized it, but I guess that's right. Talking with you makes it much clearer to me."

"Talking has shed light for all of us, Ray. No one is trying to talk you into the surgery. You just need to think about what is motivating your decision. You need to consider the ramifications of this decision. You now have more information. The final decision is yours."

Lest Sarah and I forget it is important to 'let go of the outcome,' I cautioned that he might still refuse surgery. Sarah called the next day to say that Ray had been discharged.

Several months later, Sarah called to tell me Ray was asking to see me. I thought "Oh no, he's had a heart attack." He actually stopped by to see both of us. When he left the hospital, he had done a lot more thinking. He knew 'in his heart' that he really wanted a divorce. When he spoke of it, his wife was of the same mind. They remained good friends and saw one another when visiting their children. He had moved to his special place and chosen to have heart surgery at a hospital in that area. When he looked into my eyes, I knew he was thanking me for helping him save his own life. ∎

Donna Ehrenreich, MN, RN, CS
1979

197

JOSH

I was the head nurse of a cardiac surgery intensive care unit at a 'fledgling' tertiary care center in suburban New York. The open-heart surgery program was new and so my days were often 10 to 16 hours long.

It was about 7 pm and I was in my office, putting on my coat, lamenting the fact that so often I arrived at work in the dark and went home in the dark. One of the surgeons appeared in my doorway and told me that he would be operating on a 15-year-old boy in the morning to repair a congenital heart defect. He had just come from obtaining consent for the surgery from Josh and his parents. He said that Josh had been withdrawn and seemed 'terrified.' I removed my coat and went up to Josh's room, knowing that he would be less frightened the next day in the ICU if he saw a familiar face and heard a familiar voice.

For the next half-hour, I answered the questions that Josh's parents had forgotten to ask the surgeon. Josh listened intently but quietly. I directed the parents to the coffee shop and told them I would stay with Josh while they got something to eat or drink, since they had a long night ahead of them. Josh and I spent the next hour talking about 'everything'—

his school, his older brother, his girlfriend, and his fears about the impending surgery. I noticed a guitar sitting in the corner of his room and, since he had no roommate, I closed the door and asked him to play something for me. To my surprise and delight he played an old favorite song of mine 'You've Got A Friend.'

I saw my new buddy, Josh, early the next morning in the operating room and stayed with him until he fell asleep from the anesthesia. I walked back to my unit to help the nurses prepare for his post-operative admission. Josh died in the operating room that evening. The surgeon and surgical team, faced with problems impossible to predict, fought valiantly for many, many hours to save Josh's life. They were all devastated and exhausted and, finally, they had to accept his death. The surgeon came to the unit to tell me. When I saw his face, I knew I had to be with him when he told Josh's family.

I located them and sequestered them in a private, quiet room. The surgeon met us there. He expressed his sorrow and delivered the awful news. Josh's father and brother sat still in shocked, stunned silence. His mother was far more demonstrative in her grief. She screamed and cried and moaned as she threw herself to the floor. I knelt down beside her, rubbed her back, and thought to myself how profoundly inadequate I felt as I told her how sorry I was for her loss. After some time, she turned and asked me if he had suffered any pain before he died. I assured her that he had been asleep, under anesthesia, throughout the ordeal. She then thanked me for spending so much time with Josh the previous evening. She told me that after I left, Josh had fallen asleep and had slept peacefully through the night.

Later, as I walked back to the ICU, I noted the darkness outside. There are times when I need some extra motivation to offer support and comfort to a patient because I'm so busy or tired or stressed. I close my eyes for a moment and I can almost see Josh softly strumming his guitar and hear his sweet rendition of 'You've Got A Friend.' ∎

Christine Yano, RN, CCP
1979

MAUREEN

Hospice is like Lamaze, but at the other end of life. For the hospice nurse, it can be rewarding to help the patient die *their* way and be free from pain and suffering, surrounded by family and loved ones. For years, as a hospice nurse I handled emergencies of patients in their homes during the night and on weekends. Now as an RN liaison, I connect hospice with the community, telling the story that hospice is not about death—it is about life.

This story is different from any other, because it is about both. Maureen had just found out she was pregnant. Two weeks later, she was informed that she had cancer. If she chose to have aggressive treatment to save her own life, the baby would die. Instead, she chose life for her unborn child and refused treatment.

Several days before Christmas, she was induced into labor and gave birth to a 3-pound baby boy. When the hospice nurse came into the hospital room, shortly after delivery, she found Maureen quietly weeping with the bundled-up baby boy lying across her chest. Maureen had been given weeks left to live. The hospice nurse commented on how overwhelming it was to see life and death so close together.

The baby needed to stay in the hospital to be monitored, and Maureen would be discharged home. She would spend her last days with her husband and her two children, ages 2 and 4.

Joe had no money to buy Christmas gifts for their children. The story quickly spread among the hospice staff. A collection was taken up and $700.00 was collected within 24 hours. Food was donated by a local grocery store. Gifts were purchased and wrapped for every member of the family.

On Christmas Eve, the hospice minivan was loaded up to the max. It wasn't Santa who was coming to visit. It was hospice angels trying to ease some of the burden and pain for one special family.

The hospice ambulance company offered to transport Maureen back to the hospital, at no charge to see her baby one last time—but she was too sick to make the trip.

Upon hearing this, the local hospital offered to transport the baby in a portable incubator with a private RN in *their* ambulance, at no charge, to see the mother. All they needed to know was 'when to make this all happen.' The father said "Tomorrow, on Christmas . . . so we can have a family picture together." Maureen said "No, I need to see my baby today." She lived another 2 weeks and was able to hold her baby yet one more time.

Nurses will do whatever it takes to help. Nurses want patients and their families to know that they're never alone and that we really do care. ∎

---

an Barber Grinzi, RN Liaison
᠎7

200

CONTRIBUTORS

(Vignette page number[s] follow author's address.)

Susan Allison, MS, RN, CS, CETN
Wound, Ostomy, Continence Clinical
Nurse Specialist
Armonk, NY
(70, 116)

**Diane J. Angelini, EdD, RN, CNM,
   CNAA, FACNM**
Clinical Assistant Professor
Brown University Medical School
   of Medicine
Director, Nurse-Midwifery Section
Women and Infants' Hospital
Providence, RI
(125)

Rosze Barrington, MS, RN, ANP, CS
Adult Nurse Practitioner
Employee Occupational Health Services
Abbott Northwestern Hospital
Allina Health System
Minneapolis, MN
(92, 154)

Carol Bartolotti, MPA, RN, C
New City, NY
(183)

Karen Bauer, MS, RN
Visiting Nurses Association
Thornwood, NY
(55, 162)

Roberta Lee Block, MS, RN, CS
Geriatric Clinical Nurse Specialist
Instructor, California State Dominguez Hills
Legal Nurse Consultant
San Francisco, CA
(182)

Perri Jane Bomar, PhD, RN
Associate Dean and Professor
University of North Carolina at
   Wilmington School of Nursing
Wilmington, NC
(143)

Ramita Bonadonna, MSN, RN, CS
Psychiatric Consultation Liaison Nurse
Medical University of South Carolina
Charleston, SC
(146)

**Mary Ann Bord-Hoffman, MN, MA,
   RN, AOCN**
Clinical Nurse Specialist, Oncology
Veterans Affairs Palo Alto Health Care
   System
Palo Alto, CA
(137)

Jill Bormann, PhD, RN, CS
Project Coordinator, Clinical Research
Assistant Clinical Professor
University of California San Diego
San Diego, CA
Nursing Instructor, University of Phoenix
(124, 181)

Deborah Boyle, MSN, RN, AOCN
Inova Fairfax Hospital
Falls Church, VA
(81)

Rachel Briston-Griffon, BSN, RN
Allegheny General Hospital
Pittsburgh, PA
(113)

Marlys Bueber, MN, RN, CNS
Huilongguan Hospital
Beijing
Peoples Republic of China
(59, 129)

Lori Burnell, MSN, RN
Nurse Executive
Poway, CA
(60)

Rita Callahan, MA, RN
Nurse Educator
Scripps Home Health Care Services
San Diego, CA
(13, 78)

Jan Cipkala-Gaffin, MN, RN, CS
Psychiatric Clinical Nurse Specialist
Pittsburgh, PA
(69)

Judy Cohen, Phd, RN
Associate Professor
University of Vermont School of Nursing
South Burlington, VT
(74)

Santa J. Crisall, MA, RN, C
New York, NY
(135)

Sharon Henchal Deeny, MSN, RN,
  CCRN
Inova Fairfax Hospital
Falls Church, VA
(141)

Kathleen Ann DeGrazia, BSN, MA, RN
Dongzhimenwai
Beijing
Peoples Republic of China
(14)

Debbie DenBoer, BSN, RN, CGRN
Charge Nurse, Endoscopy Department
Scripps Memorial Hospital
La Jolla, CA
(9)

Judith DePalma, MSN, RN
Director, Nursing Research
Allegheny General Hospital
Pittsburgh, PA
(102)

Jürgen Deutzer, RN
San Diego, CA
(4)

Deborah Dunne, MSN, RN, MBA
Administrator
Scripps Hospital East County
El Cajon, CA
(101)

Donna Ehrenreich, MN, RN, CS
Psychiatric Clinical Nurse Specialist
Boise, ID
(64, 196)

Barbara Fendorak, RN
West Nyack, NY
(33)

Rick Ferri, PhD, RN, ANP, ACRN
Provincetown, MA
(165)

Maggie Finch, MA, RN
Deputy Director of Nursing
Westchester Medical Center
Valhalla, NY
(72)

Jacquelyn H. Flaskerud, PhD, RN, FAAN
Professor, UCLA School of Nursing
Los Angeles, CA
(134)

Ann K. Frantz, BSN, RN
Independent Healthcare Consultant
Pontiac, MI
(168)

Kelly Gaul, MSN, RN, CS
Psychiatric Consultation Liaison Nurse
Denver, CO
(47, 142, 195)

Sue Gemar Lloyd, RN
Scripps Mercy Hospital
San Diego, CA
(77)

Renee C. Grieger, BSN, RN
Inova Health System
Falls Church, VA
(123)

Joan Barber Grinzi, RN Liaison
San Diego Hospice
San Diego, CA
(200)

Sandra S. Gunderson Goldsmith, MSN, RN, CS
Clinical Care Coordinator
Crisis Recovery Unit
San Diego County Psychiaric Hospital
San Diego, CA
(5, 177)

Kathleen P. Hanna, EdD, RN, CRNA
Program Director, Clinical and Didactic
Instructor
Pennsylvania Hospital Nurse Anesthesia
Program
Philadelphia, PA
(100)

Susan H. Harris, DNSc, RN
Special Assistant to President
National University
La Jolla, CA
(179)

Pat Harris-Murray, MN, RN
Tucson, AZ
(176)

Hazel M. Harrison, RN, CCRN
Spring Valley, CA
(30)

Cindy Hess, RN, CNOR II
Sharp Memorial Hospital
San Diego, CA
(174)

Marguerite McMillan Jackson, PhD, RN, FAAN
Administrative Director, Nursing Research
and Education and Epidemiology Unit
University of California San Diego
Medical Center
Associate Clinical Professor of Family
and Preventive Medicine
University of California San Diego
School of Medicine
San Diego, CA
(12)

Cindy Jones, MS, RN, AOCN
Veterans Affairs, San Diego Health Care
System
San Diego, CA
(80)

Mary Lou Helfrich Jones, PhD, RN, CNAA
Assistant Operating Officer
Women's Services
Duke University Medical Center
Durham, NC
(15)

Angela C. Joseph, MSN, RN, CURN
Urology/SCI Nurse Coordinator
Veterans Affairs, San Diego Healthcare
System
San Diego, CA
(38)

Jim Kane, MN, RN, CS, CNAA
Director, Psychiatric Liaison Services
Scripps Mercy Hospital
San Diego, CA
(51, 144)

Ann Kelly, MSN, RN, CS
Patient Education Coordinator
San Diego Veterans Affairs Healthcare
System
San Diego, CA
(26, 75)

Joyce Marth Knestrick, PhD (c), FNP, RN
Wheeling Health Right
Wheeling Jesuit University
Wheeling, WV
(31)

Mary Kodiath, MS, RNC, ANP
Poway, CA
(86)

Kathleen Krebs, BSN, RN
Manager, Integrated Medicine Program
Allegheny General Hospital
Pittsburgh, PA
(152)

Jill Kunkel, RN
Clinical Research Nurse
University of California, San Diego
Treatment Center
San Diego, CA
(109, 170)

Maria Lasater, MSN, RN, CCRN
Clinical Applications Specialist
Cardiodynamics International Corporation
San Diego, CA
(120)

Mary Anne LaTorre, MA, RN, CNS
Counselor, Educator, Holistic Health
Practitioner
Owner, Inner Visions
Exton, PA
(35, 127)

Susan M. Leininger, MSN, RN
Advanced Practice Nurse
Allegheny General Hospital
Pittsburgh, PA
(138)

Joan Such Lockhart, PhD, RN, CORLN
Associate Professor & Chair,
Undergraduate Nursing Program
Duquesne University School of Nursing
Pittsburgh, PA
(16)

Mary Loftus, BSN, RN, CDE
Director, Patient and Community
Education
Nyack Hospital
Nyack, NY
(139)

Catherine Flynn Loveridge, PhD, RN, PN
Professor
School of Nursing
San Diego State University
San Diego, CA
(76, 85)

Barbara E. McGurgan, MSN, RN, CCRN
Clinical Education Specialist,
Cardiovascular Surgery
Allegheny General Hospital
Pittsburgh, PA
(7, 90)

Renee P. McLeod, MSN, RN, CPNP
Scripps Mercy Pediatric Clinic
San Diego, CA
(40, 50, 63)

Jane Milazzo, MS, RN, LPN, CS
Psychiatric Clinical Nurse Specialist
Valhalla, NY
(97)

Pamela A. Minarik, MS, RN, CS, FAAN
Associate Professor
Yale University School of Nursing
Psychiatric Consultation Liaison
   Nurse Specialist
Yale New Haven Hospital
New Haven, CT
(106)

Marlene Nadler Moodie, MSN, RN, CS
Clinical Nurse Specialist—
Behavioral Health
Scripps Mercy Hospital
San Diego, CA
(19)

Kate Morse, MS, RN, ANP-C, ACNP, CCRN
Advanced Practice Nurse —
   Cardiothoracic Surgery
Scripps Mercy Hospital
San Diego, CA
(39)

Jane Bryant Neese, PhD, RN, CS
Assistant Professor, Department of
  Family and Community Nursing
College of Nursing and Health
  Professions
University of North Carolina at
  Charlotte
Charlotte, NC
  (57, 172)

Margaret A. Nelson, MSN, RN
Education Coordinator
Inova Health System
Falls Church, VA
  (153)

Linda Newton, RN, MN, CPMHN (C)
Psychiatric Consultation Liaison
  Nurse
Health Sciences Centre
Winnipeg, Manitoba
  (163)

Donna Nolten, MN, RN, C, CNA
Scripps Corporate
San Diego, CA
  (67, 184, 191)

Kiyoka Nozue, PhD, RN, PLCNS
Okazawa-CH056
Hodogaya-Ku, Yokohoma-City
Japan
  (166)

Kelly Jane O'Hara, RN, BSN, CEN
Garnerville, NY
  (18)

E'Louise Ondash, RN
North County Times
Escondido, CA
  (131)

Gale Osborn, MA, RN, C
Partial Hospital Charge Nurse
Behavioral Health Outpatient
Scripps Mercy Hospital
San Diego, CA
  (95, 147)

Annetta Parente, LPN
Minnesota, WI
  (186)

Mickey L. Parsons, PhD, RN
Tucson, AZ
  (36)

Luc R. Pelletier, MSN, RN, CS, CPHQ
Health Care Consultant
Editor, *Journal for Healthcare Quality*
Washington, DC
  (83, 175)

Mary Prehoden, RN
San Diego, CA
  (104)

Michelle Prior, MSN, RN
Pediatric Advanced Practice Nurse
Allegheny General Hospital
Pittsburgh, PA
  (108)

Susan Quaal, PhD, APRN, CVS,
  CCRN
Department of Veterans Affairs
  Medical Center
Salt Lake City, UT
  (34)

Patricia Reddish, MSN, RN, CS
Psychiatric Clinical Nurse Specialist
New York, NY
  (24, 53, 188)

Christine M. Reed, RN, CNOR
Administrator
HealthSouth Center for Surgery
  of Encinitas
Encinitas, CA
  (187)

Barbara Riegel, DNSc, RN, CS, FAAN
Professor, School of Nursing
San Diego State University
Clinical Research Sharp Health Care
San Diego, CA
  (149)

Ann Robinette, MS, RN, CS
Psychiatric Clinical Nurse Specialist
Glenville, NC
  (21)

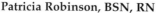

Patricia Robinson, BSN, RN
Orthopedic Patient Nurse Liaison
Chair, Mercy Outreach Surgical Team
Scripps Mercy Hospital
San Diego, CA
    (98, 158)

Christine A. Rodighiero, RN
Post Anesthesia Care Unit
Scripps Memorial Hospital
La Jolla, CA
    (32, 159)

Joanne Santangelo, MSN, RN
Family Nurse Practitioner
University of California San Diego
    Treatment Center
San Diego, CA
    (93)

Martha Scott, MSN, RN
San Diego, CA
    (99)

Edward L. Seefried, RN
Research Nurse
University of California San Diego
AIDS Treatment Center
San Diego, CA
    (156)

Marilyn J. Shirk, MSN, RN
Mental Health Clinical Nurse Specialist
Los Angeles, CA
    (192)

Kathy Lynn Springer, RN
Scripps Mercy Hospital
San Diego, CA
    (11)

Karen Stanley, MS, RN, CS
Psychiatric Clinical Nurse Specialist
Mt. Pleasant, SC
    (190)

Jaynelle F. Stichler, DNSc, RN
Principal-Healthcare Division
The Stichler Group, Inc.
San Diego, CA
    (87)

Karen A. Tarolli, BSN, RN
Clinical Research Nurse Coordinator—
    Cardiology
Allegheny General Hospital
Pittsburgh, PA
    (121)

James P. Veronesi, MSN, RN, CEN
Clinical Supervisor
Allegheny General Hospital
Pittsburgh, PA
    (151)

Marlys Vespe, MSN, RN
Medical Surgical
Clinical Nurse Specialist
Scripps Mercy Hospital
San Diego, CA
    (42)

Carmen Germaine Warner, MSN, RN, FAAN
Nurse Consultant
Editor, *Topics in Emergency Medicine*
San Diego, CA
    (44, 118)

Rose Weintraub, RN
Patient Representatives Manager
Abbott Northwestern Hospital
Minneapolis, MN
    (43)

Margo Foltz Wilson, MS, RN, CS, CGP
Psychiatric Liaison
Psychiatric Evaluation and Triage Team
Scripps Hospitals
San Diego, CA
    (27, 140)

Christine Yano, RN, CCP
Cardiothoracic Surgery
Westchester County Health
    Care Corporation
Westchester, NY
    (199)

Rick Zoucha, DNSc, RN, CS
Assistant Professor
Duquesne University School of Nursing
Pittsburgh, PA
    (89)